A Comprehensive Guide to Nanoparticles in Medicine

Authored by

Rituparna Acharya
Institute of Management Study
Kolkata
India

A Comprehensive Guide to Nanoparticles in Medicine

Author: Rituparna Acharya

ISBN (Online): 978-1-68108-835-8

ISBN (Print): 978-1-68108-836-5

ISBN (Paperback): 978-1-68108-837-2

need for a court order if at any point you breach any terms of this License Agreement. In no event will any delay or failure by Bentham Science Publishers in enforcing your compliance with this License Agreement constitute a waiver of any of its rights.

3. You acknowledge that you have read this License Agreement, and agree to be bound by its terms and conditions. To the extent that any other terms and conditions presented on any website of Bentham Science Publishers conflict with, or are inconsistent with, the terms and conditions set out in this License Agreement, you acknowledge that the terms and conditions set out in this License Agreement shall prevail.

Bentham Science Publishers Ltd.
Executive Suite Y - 2
PO Box 7917, Saif Zone
Sharjah, U.A.E.
Email: subscriptions@benthamscience.net

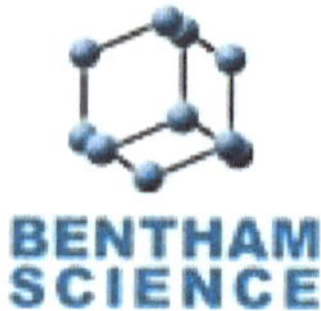

CONTENTS

FOREWORD i

PREFACE ii
CONSENT FOR PUBLICATION iii
CONFLICT OF INTEREST iii

ACKNOWLEDGEMENTS iv

CHAPTER 1 INTRODUCTION OF NANOPARTICLES IN MEDICINE 1
INTRODUCTION 1
REFERENCES 4

CHAPTER 2 THE PROCEDURE OF SYNTHESIS OF NANOPARTICLES USED AS DIAGNOSTICS AND THERAPY AVAILABLE TILL DATE 7
INTRODUCTION 7
CHEMICAL METHODS OF NANOPARTICLE SYNTHESIS 8
Co-Precipitation 8
Sol-Gel Method 10
Microemulsion Method 11
Hydrothermal Technique 13
Polyol Synthesis 14
Microwave Assisted Synthesis 14
Chemical Vapor Deposition (CVD) & Chemical Vapor Synthesis (CVS) 15
Plasma Enhanced Chemical Vapor Deposition (PECVD) 16
PHYSICAL METHODS OF NANOPARTICLE SYNTHESIS 17
High Energy Ball Milling 17
Inert Gas Condensation 18
Physical Vapor Deposition 19
Laser Pyrolysis 20
Flame Spray Pyrolysis 21
Electrospraying 21
Melt Blending 22
BIO-ASSISTED METHODS 23
Biogenic Synthesis Using Microorganisms 23
Biogenic Synthesis Using Bio-molecules as the Templates 24
Biogenic Synthesis Using Plant Extracts 25
CONCLUSION 25
REFERENCES 28

CHAPTER 3 RECENT PROGRESS OF NANOPARTICLES USED IN THE DIAGNOSIS OF DIFFERENT TYPES OF DISEASES 39
INTRODUCTION 39
NANOPARTICLE BASED DIAGNOSIS 40
Emission-Based Detection 40
Fluorescence-Based Detection 41
Colorimetric Detection 45
Microarray Detection 46
Magnetic-Based Detection 47
Magnetic Resonance Imaging (MRI) 47
Nuclear Magnetic Resonance (NMR) 48
Electrochemical-Based Detection 49
Gold Nanoparticles 49

Silver Nanoparticle 49
Quantum Dot Nanoparticles 49
Cerium oxide nanoparticles (CeO2 NPs) 50
Mercury Selenide Nanoparticles (HgSe NPs) 50
Copper-based Nanoparticles (CuNPs) 50
Plasmonics-Based Detection 50
Surface-Enhanced Raman Scattering (SERS) 50
Surface-Enhanced Infrared Absorption (SEIRA) 51
Metal Enhanced Fluorescence (MEF) 51
CONCLUSION 52
REFERENCES 53

CHAPTER 4 DRUG DELIVERY THROUGH NANOPARTICLE IN TREATMENT OF DISEASES 57
INTRODUCTION 57
CHARACTERISTICS OF NANOPARTICLE FOR THE FABRICATION OF DRUG DELIVERY VEHICLE 58
Size of Nanoparticles 58
Surface Property of Nanoparticles 59
Drug Loading and Release From the Nanoparticle 59
APPLICATION OF NANOPARTICLES IN DRUG DELIVERY 59
Cancer Therapy 59
HIV and AIDS Treatment 60
Nutraceutical Delivery Through Nanoparticles 60
NANOCARRIERS FOR DRUG DELIVERY 60
Organic Polymer Based Nanocarriers 61
Chitosan 61
Alginate 61
Xanthan Gum 62
Cellulose 62
Liposomes 62
Dendrimers 62
Inorganic Nanoparticles 63
Carbon Nanotubes 63
Gold Nanoparticles 64
Quantum Dots 64
Superparamagnetic Iron-Oxide Nanoparticles 64
Silica Nanoparticles 64
CONCLUSION 65
REFERENCES 65

CHAPTER 5 NANOPARTICLE-DNA CONJUGATE: THE TREATMENT AND DIAGNOSTIC OPTION FOR FUTURE CURE OF DISEASES 70
INTRODUCTION 70
DNA-NANOPARTICLE CONJUGATES IN NANOMEDICINE 71
DNA-Gold Nanoparticle Conjugate 72
Binding Between DNA and Gold Nanoparticle 72
Application of DNA-Gold Nanoconjugate in Nucleic Acid Detection 72
Application of DNA-Gold Nanoparticle for Colorimetric Detection of Miscellaneous Analytes 73
Application of DNA-Gold Nanoconjugate for Gene And Drug Delivery 73
DNA-Silver Conjugate Nanoparticle 73

Plasmonic Application of DNA-Silver Nanoconjugate 74
DNA-Magnetic Nanoparticle 74
Gene Therapy 74
Fluorescence Detection Method 74
DNA-Platinum and Palladium Nanoparticles 74
Electrochemical Detection 75
DNA Detection in Chip Based Microarrays 75
DNA-Quantum Dots Nanoconjugate 75
Biosensing Application 75
Gene Delivery and Therapeutics 75
DNA-Carbon Nanotubes 76
Chemical Biosensors 76
Detection of Nucleic Acid Sequence 76
Biological Transporters 76
DNA-Chitosan Nanoparticle 77
Gene Therapy 77
CONCLUSION 77
REFERENCES 78

CHAPTER 6 NANOPARTICLE CONJUGATED WITH SIRNA FOR TREATMENT OF DIFFERENT TYPES OF DISEASE CONDITIONS 83
INTRODUCTION 83
siRNAs as Potential Therapeutics 84
CHALLENGES IN DELIVERY OF siRNA 84
Administrative Barrier 85
Vascular Barrier 85
Cellular Barriers 85
Immune Response and Safety 85
OVERCOMING THE MAJOR BARRIERS FOR SIRNA DELIVERY 86
Intravenous Administration 86
Optimization of the Size of the siRNA Nanocarrier 86
Endocytosis of siRNA-nanoparticle Conjugate 86
Overcoming the Immune Response 87
NANOPARTICLE IN SIRNA THERAPY 87
siRNA-silica Based Nanoconjugate 87
siRNA-metal and Metal Oxide Nanoconjugates 88
siRNA-carbon Based Nanoconjugates 89
siRNA-dendrimer Nanoconjugates 90
siRNA-polymer Nanoconjugate 90
siRNA-Cyclodextrin Nanoconjugate 91
siRNA-lipid Based Nanoconjugates 91
siRNA-hydrogel Nanoconjugate 92
siRNA-quantum Dot Nanoconjugate 92
CONCLUSION 93
REFERENCES 94

CHAPTER 7 shRNA-NANOPARTICLE CONJUGATE AS A THERAPEUTIC OPTION 100
INTRODUCTION 100
shRNA-NANOPARTICLE CONJUGATES 101
Inorganic Nanoconjugates 101
Organic Nanoconjugates 102
Polymeric Nanoconjugates 103

Other Nanoparticle Conjugates 105
CONCLUSION 107
REFERENCES 108

CHAPTER 8 miRNA AND NANOPARTICLE CONJUGATE AS A FUTURE THERAPEUTIC APPROACH 117
INTRODUCTION 117
Tissue Specific Expression 118
Circulation miRNAs 118
THERAPEUTIC APPROACHES USING MIRNAS 119
miRNA Suppression Therapy 119
miRNA Replacement Therapy 120
CHALLENGES IN mIRNA BASED THERAPIES 120
Instability within Blood Vascular System 121
Reduced Intracellular Delivery 121
Off Target Effects 121
NANOPARTICLE ASSISTED mIRNA DELIVERY 121
Inorganic Nanoparticle Based Delivery of miRNA and Anti-miRNA 122
Gold Nanoconjugate 122
Graphine Nanoconjugate 122
Mesoporous Silica Nanoconjugate 122
Quantum Dot Nanoconjugate 123
Magnetic Nanoconjugate 123
Organic Nanoparticle Based Delivery of miRNA and Anti-miRNA 123
Chitosan Based Nanoconjugate 123
Lipid/liposome Based Nanoconjugate 123
Protein or Peptide Based Nanoconjugate 124
Aptamers Nanoconjugate 124
Polymeric Nanoparticle Based Delivery of miRNA and Anti-miRNA 124
Polyethyleneimine Nanoconjugate 125
Dendrimer Nanoconjugate 125
PLGA Based Nanoconjugate 125
Cyclodextrin Nanoconjugate 126
CHALLENGES WITH RNA NANOTECHNOLOGY 126
Challenge in RNA Structure Prediction 126
Stability of the Nanoconjugate 126
In Vivo Half-life and Retention Time of the Nanoconjugate 126
Limited Carrying Capacity of the Nanoparticle 127
Scaling Up of the Conjugate 127
Hurdles in Endosomal Escape of the Payload 127
CONCLUSION 127
REFERENCES 128

CHAPTER 9 NANOPARTICLE IMMUNOTHERAPY 135
INTRODUCTION 135
NANOPARTICLES IN IMMUNOTHERAPY 136
Antigen Delivery by Nanoparticles 136
Adjuvant Delivery by Nanoparticles 136
Co-delivery of Antigen and Adjuvant by Nanoparticles 137
Activation of Dendritic Cells by Nanoparticles 137
Change of Tumor Microenvironment by Nanoparticles 138
Delivery of Antibodies by Nanoparticles 138

Gene Delivery by Nanoparticles 139
Cytokine Delivery by Nanoparticles 139
Therapeutic Cellular Engineering by Nanoparticles 140
Overcoming Immunosuppression by Nanoparticles 140
Immune Check Point Inhibition by Nanoparticles 140
Induced Immunogenic Cell Death by Nanoparticles 141
TYPES OF NANOPARTICLES IN IMMUNOTHERAPY 142
Inorganic Nanoparticles 142
Organic Nanoparticles 143
Polymeric Nanoparticles 143
CONCLUSION 143
REFERENCES 144

CHAPTER 10 NANOPARTICLE VACCINES 152
INTRODUCTION 152
CHARACTERIZATION OF NANOVACCINES 153
Size 153
Surface Charge 154
Shape 154
Hydrophobicity 154
Surface Modification 155
NANOPARTICLE VACCINES 155
Inorganic Nanoconjugates 156
Organic Nanoconjugates 156
Polymeric Nanoconjugates 157
IMMUNE STIMULATOR USING NANOCARRIER 157
Cytokines 157
Toll Like Receptor Agonists 158
Nucleic Acids 158
CONCLUSION 158
REFERENCES 159

CHAPTER 11 CONCLUSION 167

GLOSSARY 171

SUBJECT INDEX 175

FOREWORD

Drug administration without any side effects is The need of the hour in today's research. Nanotechnology has emerged as a tool for the creation of nanoparticles that are less than 100nm in size. These nanomaterials have a wide variety of applications in medicine for diagnostic and imaging purposes, and also in targeted drug delivery and gene delivery. Targeted drug delivery may reduce the side effects of the drugs and is the priority research area in nanotechnology. On the other hand, gene deliveries in the form of DNA/siRNA/shRNA/miRNAs are the burning issue in nanomaterial and technology. The invention of immunotherapy and vaccines is the priority of today's research.

However, even though excellent nanocarriers have been invented, still there are many areas that need to be resolved before their clinical application. How to improve these nanomaterials for practical application in the treatment of diseases is the main question in research today? How can the gene delivery system be improved to make it free from off-target side effects? These were the few questions that are kept in mind while writing this book.

This book written by Dr. Rituparna Acharya is of interest not only for pharmacy students but also for the researchers and students of nanotechnology, biology and the researchers of drug delivery and medical imaging. The book "A Comprehensive Guide to Nanoparticles in Medicine" links academic knowledge with the research in nanomaterials.

Jui Chakraborty
CSIR-Central Glass and Ceramic Research Institute India
Kolkata
India

PREFACE

This book is intended to focus on the delivery of nanoparticles in several disease conditions. The synthesis methods of these nanoparticles are unique in their approach. The novel diagnostic procedures through nanoparticles are used to identify diseases in humans. The delivery of drugs conjugated with nanoparticles can optimize the dosage level and help in delivering the same to the intended target organ. Various types of nanoparticles, including the organic, inorganic and polymeric in structure are under investigation to deliver them for diagnostic and therapeutic purposes. This book covers various nanoparticle conjugates, for example, when the nanoparticle is conjugated with drugs or DNAs or siRNAs, or shRNAs or miRNAs. All aspects of immunotherapy and vaccination strategy are also included in this book. Up to date information about the nanoparticles used in medicine is the intention of the book.

In particular, chapter 1 discusses the introduction of nanoparticles that are extensively used in medicine. It gives an overview of the proceeding chapters in a consistent manner.

Chapter 2 focuses on the synthesis method of the nanoparticles that are used in medicine. It discusses the advantages and drawbacks of the synthesis methods in detail along with the characteristics and production methods in a step-by-step manner.

Chapter 3 discusses the diagnostic procedures using nanoparticles along with their advantages, disadvantages and their applications in different fields of medicines.

Chapter 4 gives an overview of the characteristics of the nanoparticles that help them to deliver the drug to the target site, their application in medicine and this chapter also discusses the wide variety of nanoparticles that are used for this purpose.

DNA-nanoparticle conjugate is the subject of chapter 5 that presents an overview of the different types of nanoconjugates used in the treatment and diagnosis of disease conditions.

Chapter 6 describes the challenges in the delivery of siRNAs and methods of overcoming those challenges using nanoconjugates. We described the advantages and disadvantages of using siRNA-nanoparticle conjugates in medicine.

shRNA-nanoparticle conjugates are the topic of discussion of chapter 7 that describes the wide variety of nanoparticles that conjugate with shRNAs and targets specific genes for the treatment of a verity of diseases.

Chapter 8 demonstrates the therapeutic approaches using miRNAs. It discusses the challenges of using miRNA in therapeutics and the variety of nanoconjugates used in therapy.

Immunotherapy is the focus area of chapter 9. It discusses the role of nanoparticles in immunotherapy. The wide variety of nanoparticles is used for this purpose and is discussed in this chapter.

Characteristics of nanovaccines are described in chapter 10 and different types of nanoparticles used for vaccination to increase their efficacy are also described in this chapter. Nanoparticles used for immunostimulation are the focus area.

Chapter 11 is the chapter of conclusion that reviews the chapters already discussed in this book. It covers the synthesis method of nanoparticles, along with drug delivery, gene therapy, immunotherapy and vaccination strategies in short.

This book provides a comprehensive coverage of nanoparticles that are used in nanomedicines. It gives an overview of the synthesis methods, diagnostic strategies, drug delivery, gene delivery, immunotherapy and vaccination methods using nanoparticles. The goal of the author is to deliver the readers an up-to-date understanding of nanoparticles in clinical research.

CONSENT FOR PUBLICATION

Not applicable.

CONFLICT OF INTEREST

The author declares no conflict of interest, financial or otherwise.

Rituparna Acharya
Assistant Professor
Institute of Management Study
Kolkata
India

ACKNOWLEDGEMENTS

The success and final outcome of this book required a lot of guidance and assistance from my parents and I am extremely privileged to have got this all along the completion of my book.

I would like to thank my parents who helped me a lot in completing this book.

Rituparna Acharya
Assistant Professor
Institute of Management Study
Kolkata
India

CHAPTER 1

Introduction of Nanoparticles in Medicine

Abstract: Nanotechnology is a branch of science that deals with nanomaterials with a size of less than 100nm. These nanoparticles have a wide variety of applications in the field of bioimaging, biosensors, drug delivery, gene therapy, *etc.* The main advantage of using nanoparticles is that they may be fabricated as desired depending upon the area of application. The size, surface chemistry and physiochemical properties may be changed as required by following the parameters of synthesis. Nanoparticles may also help in RNAi therapy that delivers siRNA, shRNA and miRNAs to the target site. The major drawback of using these RNA molecules in their bare form is the fragile nature that makes them degradable by the enzymes in the blood vascular system. In this regard, nanoparticles protect them from degradation as they may encapsulate the RNA molecules within their structure. There are mainly three types of nanoparticles such as inorganic, organic and polymeric nanoparticles. In this book, we are intended to discuss the wide variety of nanoparticles that are used in biosensing, bioimaging, drug delivery, gene therapy, immunotherapy and vaccination.

Keywords: Bioimaging, Biological property, Biosensor, Chemical property, DNA, Electronic property, Immunotherapy, MiRNA, Nanocarrier, Nanomaterial, Nanomedicine, Nanotechnology, Nanoparticle, Optical property, Physical property, RNAi therapy, ShRNA, SiRNA, Theranostic, Vaccine.

INTRODUCTION

After tremendous research effort, a new branch of science originated, known as "Nanotechnology". The word "Nanotechnology" is the agglomeration of two different words i.e., "Nano" and "Technology". Nanotechnology deals with particles that have a size of less than 100nm. In the modern era, nanoparticles have a wide range of applications in the field of medicines, information technology, energy, environment, aerospace science, *etc.* [1 - 3]. As nanoparticles show improved characteristics in their small dimension, these nanomaterials have a vital role to play in the science of nanotechnology. Due to their outstanding physical, chemical, optical, electronic and biological properties, they open up new avenues of application in the scientific and technological field.

Rituparna Acharya

The size, shape, and physiochemical properties of the nanoparticles may be fabricated depending upon their utilization. Diverse size and surface properties make them potential for a wide variety of applications. Their properties may be tailor-made for appropriate applications. Inorganic, organic and polymeric nanoparticles [4, 5] may be used for a variety of applications such as drug delivery [6], bioimaging [7], biosensors [8], molecular tagging, food technology [9], antimicrobial coatings [10], textile manufacturing [11], quantum lasers [12], quantum computers [13], energy and environmental uses, *etc.* To obtain optimum size and physiochemical properties, the synthesis method of the nanoparticles is essential to study in detail. An appropriate synthesis method should be applied in order to get the desired size and surface property of the nanoparticle. In the present book, we will discuss the synthesis methods, for example, physical, chemical and bio-assisted methods.

Nanoparticles may be used also in the diagnosis of disease conditions [14]. Detection of biological and chemical components may be performed using nanoparticles. By the identification of genetic material and proteins in the body in the early stage of the disease makes the detection method more efficient. So, the diagnostic technique that is sensitive, selective and stable is in demand in the current scenario.

Biosensing method comprises two steps, firstly recognition and binding to the target element, secondly, the transduction of the signal of the binding event. These two components should be efficient enough for proper detection of the target molecule. Thus, the challenge is on the development of both of these recognition and transduction processes. However, the nanoparticles are developing new recognition and transduction methods for accurate detection of the target molecules [15]. Nanoparticles have several physical and chemical characteristics that make them ideal for manufacturing sensitive detection methods [16]. The unique optical, magnetic and electronic properties of the nanoparticles make them ideal for these applications. Moreover, nanoparticles may be conjugated with ligands and bio-macromolecules that help them in the detection system [17 - 20]. In this book, we will discuss the detection methods invented using nanoparticles for wide variety of disease conditions.

Nanoparticles may also be used as drug delivery vehicles to the target organ [21, 22]. This approach reduces the dosage and side effects of the drugs when used in bare form. Nanoparticles resolve the problems arising from uncontrollable release of drugs, nonspecific distribution, rapid clearance, and low bioavailability [23 - 25]. Even though a wide variety of nanocarriers is developed by scientists, still, they are associated with unwanted toxicity diminishing their use in nanomedicine. This highlights the design and engineering of the nanocarriers for their use in biotechnology [26 - 28]. In this book, we are intended to discuss the newly developed nanocarriers with application in drug delivery. We will analyze the main parameters that influence drug delivery in an optimum manner. Further, we will also analyze the challenges and limitations of the newly developed areas in drug delivery.

In recent decades, nanoparticles have received enormous attention for their extraordinary functional property in the application of diagnostic and therapeutic areas. Nanoparticles are chosen as a delivery vehicle of DNA that may help in theranostic applications. Viral vectors for the delivery of plasmid DNA have demonstrated immense immune response. Nanoparticles play a vital role in this respect.

Nanoparticle in conjugation with DNA macromolecules has several applications in the field of molecular diagnosis, biosensing and gene therapy. These approaches have the opportunity to develop low-cost and highly sensitive diagnostic procedures using DNA. The study shows that DNA-nanoparticle conjugates have promising applications in near future. This book is intended to study about the wide variety of nanoparticles and their application in diagnosis and therapy. We have specifically focused on gold, silver and carbon nanoparticles in conjugation with DNA for their application in medical biotechnology.

RNAi therapy has revealed a new avenue of the therapeutic opportunity of several diseases like cancer, genetic diseases, autoimmune diseases and viral infections. siRNAs, shRNAs and miRNAs are the three types of RNAi therapeutic options that may cure many diseases. Among them, siRNAs have entered clinical trials that are being pursued as a curative measure for several diseases. Although they are showing success, still they need to be studied in more detail for their prospective commercial success as therapeutics [29].

Another RNAi therapy is through shRNAs. shRNA-nanoparticles when conjugated together they help in treating several genetic and infectious disease conditions [30 - 36]. In this book, we will discuss the wide variety of nanoparticles that may be conjugated with shRNAs and used for the treatment of many disease conditions.

The use of miRNAs is also a type of RNAi therapy. Suppression and replacement gene therapies are the main two types of mechanisms that are used for therapeutic applications. To overcome the hurdles of using bare miRNAs, nanoparticles are used. In this book, we will discuss the nanoparticles that help in the delivery of miRNAs encapsulated or in conjugation.

Along with the use of RNAi therapy, nanoparticles are also used for immune modulation. Nanoparticles are approaching a new way of treating diseases. New functionalized capability of the nanoparticles is making them available for immunotherapy. These new materials may have the potential of application in this field. In this book, we are intended to discuss the number of immunostimulators and their conjugation with a wide variety of nanoparticles.

In vaccine delivery, live attenuated microbes, killed microbes or components of microbes are used in traditional therapy. However, live vaccines are not safe for immunocompromised individuals. Moreover, there is a wide range of infectious disease conditions where vaccines are not available. So, recent attention is given to the nanoparticles that may help in antigen delivery. Antigens may be encapsulated within the nanoparticles or may be decorated over the surface to stimulate the immune response. In this book, we will review the characteristics of nanovaccines, along with the types of nanoparticles used for vaccination and also discuss the wide variety of immunostimulators that use nanocarriers.

Overall, this book is intended to deliver facts about the nanoparticles that are used in medicine for diagnostic and therapeutic intervention.

REFERENCES

[1] Lee J, Mahendra S, Alvarez PJ. Nanomaterials in the construction industry: a review of their applications and environmental health and safety considerations. ACS Nano 2010; 4(7): 3580-90. [http://dx.doi.org/10.1021/nn100866w] [PMID: 20695513]

[2] Smith DM, Simon JK, Baker JR Jr. Applications of nanotechnology for immunology. Nat Rev Immun 2013; 13(8): 592-605. [http://dx.doi.org/10.1038/nri3488] [PMID: 23883969]

[3] Nie S, Xing Y, Kim GJ, Simons JW. Nanotechnology applications in cancer. Annu Rev Biomed Eng 2007; 9: 257-88. [http://dx.doi.org/10.1146/annurev.bioeng.9.060906.152025] [PMID: 17439359]

[4] Jong WH, De Jong WH, Borm PJA. Drug delivery and nanoparticles: applications and hazards. Int J Nanomed 2008; 3(2): 133-49. [http://dx.doi.org/10.2147/ijn.s596]

[5] Hans ML, Lowman AM. Biodegradable nanoparticles for drug delivery and targeting. Curr Opin Solid State Mater Sci 2002; 6(4): 319-27. [http://dx.doi.org/10.1016/S1359-0286(02)00117-1]

[6] Salata V. Applications of nanoparticles in biology and medicine. J Nanobiotechnol 2004; 2(1): 1-6.

[7] Coto-García AM, Sotelo-González E, Fernández-Argüelles MT, Pereiro R, *et al.* Nanoparticles as fluorescent labels for optical imaging and sensing in genomics and proteomics. Anal Bioanal Chem 2011; 399(1): 29-42. [http://dx.doi.org/10.1007/s00216-010-4330-3] [PMID: 21052647]

[8] Zeng S, Yong K-T, Roy I, Dinh X-Q, Luan F. A review on functionalized gold nanoparticles for biosensing applications. Plasmonics 2011; 6(3): 491-506. [http://dx.doi.org/10.1007/s11468-011-9228-1]

[9] Saxena N, Dwivedi P. Emerging trends of nanoparticles application in food technology: Safety

paradigms. Nanotoxicology 2009; 3(1): 10-8.

[10] Taheri S, Cavallaro A, Christo SN, *et al.* Substrate independent silver nanoparticle based antibacterial coatings. Biomaterials 2014; 35(16): 4601-9. [http://dx.doi.org/10.1016/j.biomaterials.2014.02.033] [PMID: 24630091]

[11] Becheri A, Dürr M, Lo Nostro P, Baglioni P. Synthesis and characterization of zinc oxide nanoparticles: application to textiles as UV-absorbers. J Nanopart Res 2008; 10(4): 679-89. [http://dx.doi.org/10.1007/s11051-007-9318-3]

[12] Rachkovskaya GE, Zakharevich GB, Yumashev KV, Malyarevich AM, Gaponenko MS. Glasses with lead sulfide nanoparticles for laser technologies. Glass and Ceramics 2004; 61(9): 331-3. [http://dx.doi.org/10.1023/B:GLAC.0000048704.51865.06]

[13] Gadomsky O, Kharitonov Y. Quantum computer based on activated dielectric nanoparticles selectively interacting with short optical pulses. Quantum Electronics 2007; 34(3): 249.

[14] Rosenzweig Z. Principles of Chemical and Biological Sensors. Vol. 150. Chemical Analysis: A Series of Monographs on Analytical Chemistry and Its Applications By Dermot Diamond (Dublin City University, Dublin, Ireland). John Wiley & Sons, Inc.: New York. 1998. xxvii + 334 pp. $89.00. ISBN 0-471-54619-4. Journal of the American Chemical Society. 1999 1999/07/01;121(27):6522-.

[15] Sheehan PE, Whitman LJ. Detection limits for nanoscale biosensors. Nano Letters 2005; 5(4): 803-7. [http://dx.doi.org/10.1021/nl050298x]

[16] Rosi NL, Mirkin CA. Nanostructures in biodiagnostics. Chemical Reviews 2005; 105(4): 1547-62.

[17] Alivisatos P. The use of nanocrystals in biological detection. Nat Biotechnol 2004; 22(1): 47-52. [http://dx.doi.org/10.1038/nbt927] [PMID: 14704706]

[18] Niemeyer CM. Nanoparticles, proteins, and nucleic acids: biotechnology meets materials science. Angew Chem Int Ed Engl 2001; 40(22): 4128-58. [http://dx.doi.org/10.1002/1521-3773(20011119)40:22<4128::AID-ANIE4128>3.0.CO;2-S] [PMID: 29712109]

[19] West JL, Halas NJ. Applications of nanotechnology to biotechnology commentary. Curr Opin Biotechnol 2000; 11(2): 215-7. [http://dx.doi.org/10.1016/S0958-1669(00)00082-3] [PMID: 10753774]

[20] Parak W, Gerion D, Pellegrino T, Zanchet D, Micheel C, Williams S, *et al.* Biological applications of colloidal nanocrystals. Nanotechnology 2003; 14: R15. [http://dx.doi.org/10.1088/0957-4484/14/7/201]

[21] Kawasaki ES, Player A. Nanotechnology, nanomedicine, and the development of new, effective therapies for cancer. Nanomedicine 2005; 1(2): 101-9. [http://dx.doi.org/10.1016/j.nano.2005.03.002] [PMID: 17292064]

[22] Allen TM, Cullis PR. Drug delivery systems: entering the mainstream. Science 2004; 303(5665): 1818-22. [http://dx.doi.org/10.1126/science.1095833] [PMID: 15031496]

[23] Gmeiner WH, Ghosh S. Nanotechnology for cancer treatment. Nanotechnol Rev 2015; 3(2): 111-22. [PMID: 26082884]

[24] Yu X, Trase I, Ren M, Duval K, Guo X, Chen Z. Design of nanoparticle-based carriers for targeted drug delivery. J Nanomater 2016; 1087250. [http://dx.doi.org/10.1155/2016/1087250] [PMID: 27398083]

[25] Yin J, Chen Y, Zhang Z-H, Han X. Stimuli-responsive block copolymer-based assemblies for cargo delivery and theranostic applications. Polymers 2016 8: 268. [http://dx.doi.org/10.3390/polym8070268]

[26] Siegler EL, Kim YJ, Wang P. Nanomedicine targeting the tumor microenvironment: Therapeutic strategies to inhibit angiogenesis, remodel matrix, and modulate immune responses. J Cellular

Immunotherapy 2016; 2(2): 69-78.

[27] Liu D, Yang F, Xiong F, Gu N. The smart drug delivery system and its clinical potential. Theranostics 2016; 6(9): 1306-23.
[http://dx.doi.org/10.7150/thno.14858] [PMID: 27375781]

[28] Werner M, Auth T, Beales PA, *et al.* Nanomaterial interactions with biomembranes: Bridging the gap between soft matter models and biological context. Biointerphases 2018; 13(2): 028501.
[http://dx.doi.org/10.1116/1.5022145] [PMID: 29614862]

[29] Tatiparti K, Sau S, Kashaw SK, Iyer AK. siRNA delivery strategies: a comprehensive review of recent developments. Nanomat (Basel) 2017; 7(4): 77.
[http://dx.doi.org/10.3390/nano7040077] [PMID: 28379201]

[30] Weinberg MS, Arbuthnot P. Progress in the use of RNA interference as a therapy for chronic hepatitis B virus infection. Genome Medicine. 2010; 2(4): 28.
[http://dx.doi.org/10.1186/gm149]

[31] Motavaf M, Safari S, Alavian SM. Therapeutic potential of RNA interference: a new molecular approach to antiviral treatment for hepatitis C. J Viral Hepat 2012; 19(11): 757-65.
[http://dx.doi.org/10.1111/jvh.12006] [PMID: 23043382]

[32] Xiaofei E, Stadler BM, Debatis M, Wang S, Lu S, Kowalik TF. RNA interference-mediated targeting of human cytomegalovirus immediate-early or early gene products inhibits viral replication with differential effects on cellular functions. J Virol 2012; 86(10): 5660-73.
[http://dx.doi.org/10.1128/JVI.06338-11] [PMID: 22438545]

[33] Singhania R, Khairuddin N, Clarke D, McMillan NA. RNA interference for the treatment of papillomavirus disease. Open Virol J 2012; 6(6): 204-15.
[http://dx.doi.org/10.2174/1874357901206010204] [PMID: 23341856]

[34] Vlachakis D, Tsiliki G, Pavlopoulou A, Roubelakis MG, Tsaniras SC, Kossida S. Antiviral stratagems against HIV-1 using RNA interference (RNAi) technology. Evol Bioinform Online 2013; 9: 203-13.
[http://dx.doi.org/10.4137/EBO.S11412] [PMID: 23761954]

[35] Huang DT, Lu CY, Shao PL, *et al. In vivo* inhibition of influenza A virus replication by RNA interference targeting the PB2 subunit *via* intratracheal delivery. PLoS One 2017; 12(4): e0174523.
[http://dx.doi.org/10.1371/journal.pone.0174523] [PMID: 28380007]

[36] Acharya R, Hazra S, Chakraborty J. Effective cellular internalization of virion infectivity factor gene siRNA-Nanoceramic conjugate in T lymphocyte cells. Adv Sci Eng Med 2017; 9(11): 924-30.

CHAPTER 2

The Procedure of Synthesis of Nanoparticles Used as Diagnostics and Therapy Available till Date

Abstract: The ongoing research in nanotechnology has developed a number of different synthesis techniques of nanoparticles from a diverse range of materials such as metals, biological, metal oxides, ceramics, polymers, *etc.* Nanoparticles have a range of morphological, physical, chemical properties depending upon their synthesis and precursors that are important for their wide variety of applications such as biosensors, drug delivery, gene delivery, diagnostics and theragnostics. This study is intended to give a broader view of various synthesis methods available nowadays in the field of medicinal applications of nanoparticles. It also contains the advantages and shortfalls of the synthesis methods.

Keywords: Bio-templates assisted biogenesis, Chemical vapour deposition, Co-precipitation, Electrospraying, Flame spray pyrolysis, High Energy Ball Milling, Hydrothermal Technique, Inert Gas Condensation, Laser pyrolysis, Melt blending, Microemulsion, Microorganisms Assisted Biogenesis, Microwave Assisted Synthesis, Nanoparticles, Nanotechnology, Physical vapor deposition, Plant Extracts Assisted Biogenesis, Plasma enhanced chemical vapour deposition, Polyol synthesis, Sol-gel method.

INTRODUCTION

Nanotechnology is comprised of two words "nano" and "technology" that means the particles that are less than 100nm in size are synthesized in this method. The wide range of applications of this nanotechnology has led this method to emerge as a cutting edge method of the modern era. The nanomaterials developed by this procedure have unique optical, physical, chemical and biological properties that explore new avenues in the field of science and technology. To get desirable properties nanoparticles can be tailor-made, depending upon their size and shape.

Due to their small size, nanoparticles have divers' application in various fields. Depending upon the property, they can be used in medicine in the area of drug delivery, biosensor, bioimaging, molecular tagging, gene therapy, *etc.*

Rituparna Acharya

In order to use these nanoparticles in medicine, the most essential aspect is to understand the synthesis method to fabricate a desirable nanocomposite. The proper synthesis method ultimately leads to the formation of the desired size, shape, surface property of the nanoparticle. In this study, we are intended to understand and review the various synthesis methods of nanoparticles.

There are mainly two different approaches for the synthesis of nanoparticles- Top-Down Approach and Bottom-Up Approach. The top-down approach is nothing but the method by which the precursors are bulk counterparts that step by step lead to the generation of fine nanoparticles. Electron beam lithography, milling techniques, photolithography, anodization, ion and plasma etching are some of the commonly used top-down methods for the industrial production of nanoparticles. On the other hand, the bottom-up approach is nothing but the nucleation and coalescence of the molecules that lead to the formation of nanoparticles. This method is applicable for self-assembly of monomer/polymer molecules, laser pyrolysis, Co-precipitation, sol–gel processing, chemical vapor deposition, plasma or flame spraying synthesis and bio-assisted synthesis.

Generally, nanoparticle synthesis method is divided into 3 techniques *i.e.*, Chemical Method, Physical Method and Biological Method (Fig. **1**).

CHEMICAL METHODS OF NANOPARTICLE SYNTHESIS

Co-precipitations, sol-gel method, microemulsion, hydrothermal technique, polyol synthesis, microwave-assisted synthesis, chemical vapor deposition, plasma-enhanced chemical vapor deposition are the most commonly used chemical methods for nanoparticle synthesis.

Co-Precipitation

One of the chemical methods of synthesis of nanoparticles is the Co-precipitation method. In this method of synthesis, there is simultaneous occurrence of nucleation, growth, coarsening, and/or agglomeration of the nanoparticle. It is usually chosen when high purity and good stoichiometric control are needed [1]. It is a common reaction for the synthesis of nanoparticles like Fe_3O_4 [2].

Co-precipitation reaction demonstrates the following characteristics [3, 4]:

- The outcome product of this reaction is nothing but the insoluble part of the supersaturated solution.
- A wide number of small particles emerge from this reaction with large particle size distribution ranging from submicron to tens of microns if proper precautions are not taken in the nucleation stage of synthesis.

- In the Ostwald ripening procedure, the nucleation stage largely affects the size, morphology, shape and properties of the outcome product.
- Supersaturation is the ultimate condition that actually leads to the precipitation of the product.

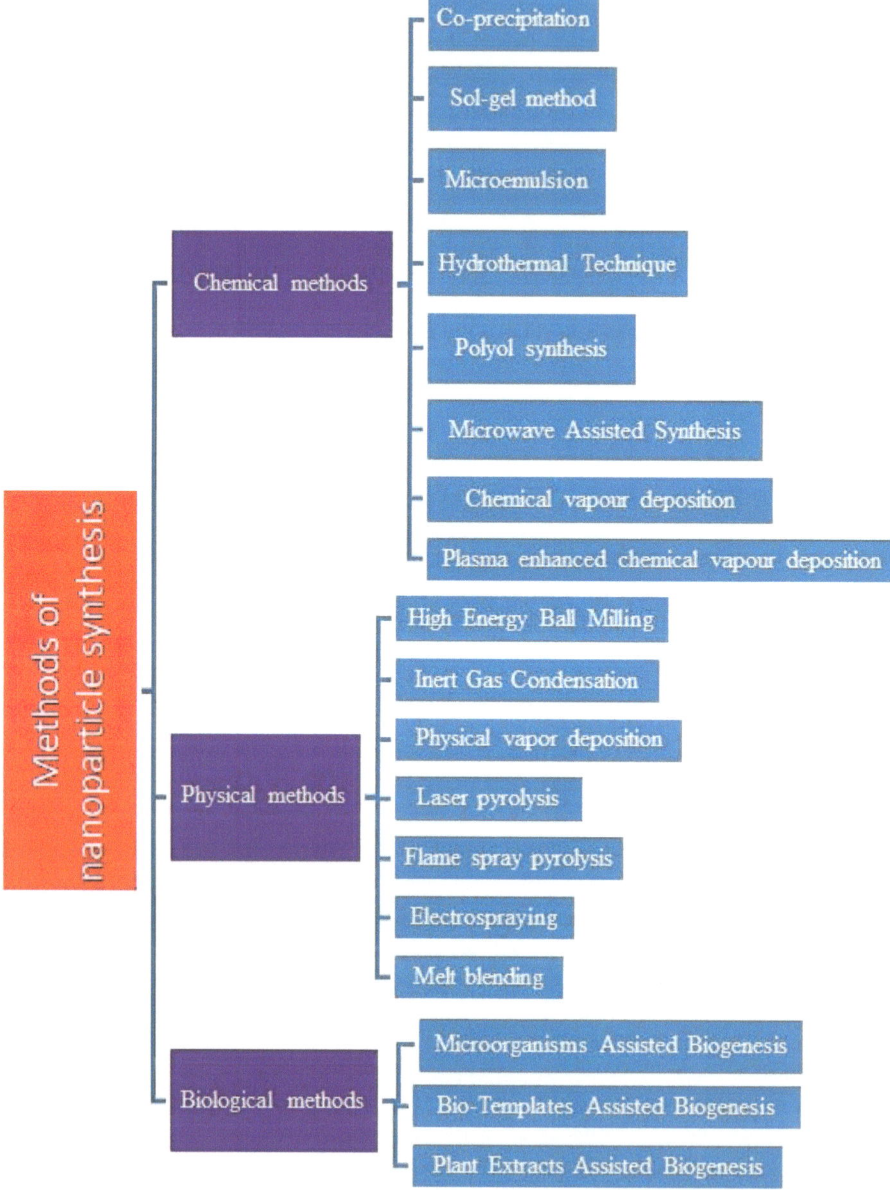

Fig. (1). Schematic diagram of the different types of nanoparticle synthesis methods.

The following stages are the methods of production of nanoparticles by the Co-precipitation method [3, 4]:

- Nanoparticles are formed from an aqueous solution or by electrochemical reduction and by decomposition of the precursor.
- Oxides are formed from the reaction.
- Metal chalconides are formed from this solution.
- Sonication or microwave is usually used to coprecipitate the product.

Co-precipitation method is a facile and convenient approach of the production of nanoparticles due to its following advantages. It also contains some disadvantages as well that are included in the following Table **1** [3 - 5]:

Table 1. Advantages and disadvantages of co-precipitation method.

Advantages	Disadvantages
Simple preparation method	Not possible for the uncharged precursors or products
It is a quick and rapid method of preparation	Impurities present in the precipitated outcome
Easy to control the particle size	Time-consuming
Easy to control the composition of the product	Toxic liquid waste
Easily available precursors	pH adjustment is necessary
Low reaction temperature	Requires proper training for production
Sustainable energy use	High capital cost
No solid waste	-
Efficient and proved technology	-
Easily usable for industry	-

Sol-Gel Method

The sol-gel method is another procedure of synthesis of nanoparticles in material chemistry. Metal oxides and mixed oxide composites are prepared by this method [6, 7]. Few steps that are hydrolysis, condensation, and drying process, lead to the development of the metal oxides by this method [8 - 10]. This procedure has better control over the surface property and texture of the material.

Followings are the characteristics of this method [3]:

- The commonly used precursors are metal alkoxides or chlorides.
- Dopes can be used like rare earth metals and organic dyes for the synthesis of the final product [11].
- The final product can be used as a casting material in the processing and manufacture of ceramics.
- Metal oxide films can also be produced by this method.

The general method of synthesis of the nanoparticle is as follows [4]:

- In the liquid phase, all the raw materials are mixed uniformly.
- Sol is prepared by hydrolysis and polycondensation reactions.
- Aging of the sols gives rise to the aggregation of colloid particles and formation of gel in three-dimensional network structures.
- By drying and sintering method nanoparticles are developed.

Sol-gel procedure is an economically feasible method with the following advantages. The disadvantages are also included in the following Table **2**:

Table 2. Advantages and disadvantages of sol-gel method.

Advantages	Disadvantages
Low temperature procedure	Long reaction time
Precursors are in molecular level	Solvents are toxic for human
Final product is homogeneous	-
High purity of the final product	-
Adjustable porosity of the final product	-
Easy to prepare	-
Simple preparation method	-
Suitable for preparing multicomponent materials with fine control	-
Enables the use of dopes in the material	-

Microemulsion Method

The term microemulsion was first coined by Schulman *et al.* in 1959 [12]. By this technique inorganic nanomaterials including metal, semiconducting metal sulphite, metal salt, metal oxide, magnetic and composite nanoparticles are synthesized. Microemulsion is nothing but a stable, transparent, homogeneous, isotropic dispersion with three phases in it *i.e.*, polar phase (usually water), non-polar phase (usually hydrocarbon liquid/oil) and surfactant phase [13].

The general characteristics of this type of synthesis method are as follows:

- The surfactant phase produces an inter-separation layer that stays between the aqueous and organic phase that reduces the interfacial tension and prevents coalescence of the droplets.
- Microemulsion leads to the development of nanoparticles that are oil-in-water or water-in-oil depending upon the surfactants used.

Following are the synthesis method of nanoparticle [14]:

- There are generally two routes of synthesis of nanoparticle: (1) One micro-emulsion method and the (2) Two microemulsion method.
- The first one is further divided into two types. The first one is the energy triggering method that requires a triggering agent to initiate the nucleation reaction in the precursor and the other method is microemulsion plus reactant method that is initiated by adding any one reactant into the microemulsion.
- In the latter method, two reactants are mixed together and the Brownian motion helps them to result in inter-micellar collisions and this leads to the mixing of the micellar components [15].
- Nucleation process within these micelle leads to the formation of nanoparticles.

Following are the advantages and disadvantages of the microemlsion method for the preparation of nanoparticles (Table 3):

Table 3. Advantages and disadvantages of microemulsion method.

Advantages	Disadvantages
Easy to prepare	Precursors are toxic in nature
Low-temperature procedure	Temperature and pH influences the stability
Stable and long self-life	Limited solubilizing capacity
Minimal agglomeration	-
High specific surface area	-
More control on size and composition	-

Hydrothermal Technique

The term 'hydrothermal' was first coined by British geologist Roderick Murchison (1792–1871). This technique is used to fabricate nanoparticles of iron oxide, metal oxide and lithium iron phosphate, *etc.*A huge amount of nanoparticles can be synthesized by this method that is optimum in size, morphology and surface chemistry [16].

Following are the characteristics of the nanoparticle that are developed by this method:

- By this method, certain nanoparticles are successfully developed that are important solids, such as superionic conductors, microporous crystals, electronically conducting solids, chemical sensing oxides, magnetic materials, complex oxide ceramic and fluorides, and luminescence phosphors.
- This method can lead to the fabrication of nanoparticles, thin films, gels, distinguished helical and chiral structures, and particularly stacking-sequence materials.
- Nanoparticles are produced from a colloidal system that comprises of two or more phases that are solid, liquid or gas states and matter *e.g.* gels and foams mixed together under controlled temperature and pressure.

Following are the synthesis method:

- Synthesis can be done by batch hydrothermal or continuous hydrothermal process.
- The former procedure can be carried out by a system with the desired ratio phases while the latter carry out a higher rate of reaction in a shorter period of time [17].

The advantages and disadvantages are as follows (Table **4**):

Table 4. Advantages and disadvantages of Hydrothermal Technique.

Advantages	Disadvantages
Inexpensive method	Needs expensive instruments
Outcome materials are soluble in a proper solvent	Safety issues
Easy to synthesis	Unobservable due to black box
Easy to control the size, shape, and crystalline structure of the final product	-

Polyol Synthesis

Polyol method is a strategy to synthesis nanoparticles with controlled size, shape and composition. It is a widely used method for the synthesis of wide range of metal based, magnetic, metal oxide and metal hybrid nanoparticles [18].

The characteristics of this synthesis method are as follows [19]:

- Polyol procedure is highly sensitive to the reaction conditions such as temperature, concentration of the precursors and chemical environment of the reaction.
- By changing these parameters the size, morphology and texture can be controlled of the final outcome product.

Synthesis method is as follows [20 - 22]:

- Synthesis method starts with the heating of polyol compounds.
- Sometimes capping agents are added.
- Reduction of the precursors and formation of nanoparticles.

Followings are the advantages and disadvantages of this synthesis method of nanoparticle (Table 5) [23]:

Table 5. Advantages and disadvantages of polyol synthesis method.

Advantages	Disadvantages
Water soluble precursors	Agglomeration effect of the nanoparticles
High boiling point	High reactivity of the final product
Instant synthesis of metals	Instability of the final product
Easy surface functionalization	-
Easy colloidal stabilization of the nanoparticle	-
Wide adaptability from low weight to high weight	-
Low temperature procedure	-

Microwave Assisted Synthesis

Microwave assisted method of synthesis of nanoparticle is a popular method.

The characteristics of this method [24]:

- Solvent of reagents absorb the microwave energy and convert into heat.
- Microwave heating is directly applied to the sample and not to the vessel.
- Depending upon the requirement the heat can be controlled that is stopped and started instantly.

Synthesis method:

- Depolarization and ionic conduction is achieved by the method of heating [25].
- When the microwave is used the dipoles of irradiated molecules in the solution try to align with the oscillating magnetic field that leads to the generation of heat.
- The amount of heat generated depends upon the frequency of the field and how fast the molecules align within the field.
- Ions also collide and oscillate within the field, and generating heat.
- The ions when collide within themselves and other ions in the solution generates large amount of heat [26].

Advantages and disadvantages are as follows (Table **6**) [27]:

Table 6. Advantages and disadvantages of Microwave Assisted Synthesis method.

Advantages	Disadvantages
Short in reaction time	Expensive equipment's are needed
Improved conversion method	Scale up is unsuitable
Final product with no contamination	Unable to monitor the reaction
Wide scope of development of the method	-
Convenient to use in case of organic synthetic method	-
Instantaneous method	-
Specific method	-
High yield	-
Easy to handle	-

Chemical Vapor Deposition (CVD) & Chemical Vapor Synthesis (CVS)

This method is usually used for the deposition of solid film in a very high temperature. The film produced by this method also contains ultra-fine particles *i.e.*, nanoparticles. Hence nanoparticles can also be prepared by this method (Table **7**).

Table 7. Advantages and disadvantages of CVD and CVS method

Advantages	Disadvantages
High percentage of doping is possible by this method	Use of very high temperature
Reduced cost	High capacity production is not possible
Higher crystal formation	Not an 'on site' procedure
Final product do not have contamination	

When the chemical vapor deposition method is modified to fabricate nanoparticles, it is known as chemical vapor synthesis.

The characteristics are as follows [28]:

- The precursors remain in three states *i.e.*, solid, liquid and gaseous.
- Doped nanoparticles can also be synthesized by using variety of precursors.
- Nucleation method ultimately leads to the formation of nanoparticles.

Synthesis steps are as follows [29]:

- Feeding of the precursors.
- Heating of the materials.
- Dilution and cooling of the materials.
- Final collection of the nanoparticles.

Plasma Enhanced Chemical Vapor Deposition (PECVD)

This procedure is used for the formation of thin film. However it is also used for the fabrication of nanoparticle.

The characteristics of Plasma enhanced chemical vapor deposition are:

- Due to the low input power and slow reaction rate monomers are formed by this method.
- Due to slow reaction rate low number of final produce are formed and high amount of precursors remain as an end product.
- Unreacted precursors react with small number of nuclei and leads to the formation of large final products.
- At higher power the unreacted species disappear and more number of nuclei can form.
- Coagulation growth can be prevented and nanoparticles can be formed by this method.

Synthesis method has following two steps [30]:

- Pre-plasma treatment
- Coating of nanoparticle array

The advantages and disadvantages are in Table **8** [31]:

Table 8. Advantages and disadvantages of PECVD method.

Advantages	Disadvantages
High deposition rate	Unstable in humidity and ageing
Low temperature	Time consuming method
Organic and inorganic materials are the precursors.	Existence of toxic and explosive gases in the plasma stream
Nanoparticles have unique chemical properties	High cost of equipment
Thermally and chemically stable	-
Solvent resistant	-

PHYSICAL METHODS OF NANOPARTICLE SYNTHESIS

High energy ball milling, inert gas condensation, physical vapor deposition, laser pyrolysis, flame spray pyrolysis, electrospraying, melt blending are the most regularly used method for the fabrication of nanoparticles. In the physical methods mechanical pressure, thermal energy, high energy radiations, electrical energy, melting, condensation, evaporation methods are used to generate nanoparticles. The physical method is proved to be less economic due to the production of abundant amount of wastes.

High Energy Ball Milling

John Benjamin in 1970 first developed the method of high energy ball milling for the synthesis of oxide dispersion strengthened alloys [32] and now a day it is being used for the fabrication of nanoparticles with various size and dimensions [33].

The characteristics of this method are as follows:

- High energy ball milling method transfers the kinetic energy of the moving balls to the milled material.
- This method leads to the rupture of the chemical bonds of the milled material

and formation of small particles that have different surface texture.

- The physical and morphological property of the resultant final nanoparticle depends upon the milling speed, media, ball-to-powder weight ratio, type of high energy ball mill, milling atmosphere and duration of milling and the material during the process.

The synthesis method includes the following steps [34]:

- The initial stage comprises of the collision of the balls and flattening of the powder particles by compressive forces.
- At the intermediate stage significant changes occur of the alloyed powders that are still not homogeneous.
- At the final stage reduction in particle size is evident. The microstructure of the particles seems to be more homogenous.
- At the completion stage the powder particles possess an extremely deformed metastable structure.

The advantages and disadvantages are as follows in Table **9** [35]:

Table 9. Advantages and disadvantages of High Energy Ball Milling method.

Advantages	Disadvantages
Can produce large quantity of nanoparticles	Difficult in classification according to the particle size
Easy to use in industries	Surface contamination
May have high production volume	Tendency to agglomerate

Inert Gas Condensation

Birringer and Gleiter group was pioneer of this method of synthesis of nanoparticles [36]. This is the primitive method of synthesis by using helium and argon the inert gases.

The characteristics of this method are as follows:

- Nanocrystalline metals and alloys are synthesized by this procedure.
- Metals are evaporated in a vacuum chamber that lose their kinetic energy and condenses in fine particles.
- These particles then grow and finally form nanocrystals.

The synthesis method is divided into 3 steps [37]:

- 1st step comprises of nucleation and growth of nanoparticle.
- 2nd step comprises of cluster collision and coalescence that leads to aggregation and formation of larger nanoparticles.
- The 3rd step comprises of the fabrication of hybrid nanoparticles that have magneto-optic bio applications.

The advantages and disadvantages are as follows in Table **10**:

Table 10. Advantages and disadvantages of Inert Gas Condensation method.

Advantages	Disadvantages
Improved control over the particle size	Very slow procedure
-	Not good for industrial application
-	Stopping agglomeration of nanoparticles are challenging

Physical Vapor Deposition

Physical vapor deposition method is a collective procedure used for the synthesis of nanoparticles and formation of thin layers from few nanometers to several micrometers [38].

The most commonly used physical vapor deposition methods are:

- Sputtering
- Electron beam evaporation
- Pulsed laser deposition
- Vacuum arc

The synthesis procedure is as follows [39]:

- Vaporization of the material from a solid source.
- Transportation of the vaporized material.
- Nucleation and growth to generate thin films and nanoparticles.

The advantages and disadvantages are as follows in Table **11** [31]:

Table 11. Advantages and disadvantages of Physical vapor deposition method.

Advantages	Disadvantages
Environment friendly	Cooling system are required
Do not require special precautions	High temperature procedure

(Table 11) cont.....

Advantages	Disadvantages
No toxic precursors	Expertise required to do
Atomic level control of chemical composition	Low deposition rate
-	Requirement of annealing time

Laser Pyrolysis

Haggerty *et al.* first developed the method of CO_2 laser pyrolysis for the synthesis of nanoparticles [40, 41]. This procedure results into the formation of various oxides, non-oxides and ternary composites.

The main characteristics of this procedure are as follows:

- At the interface of the laser beam and molecular flow of the gaseous/vapor reactants, condensable products are generated by laser induced chemical reactions.
- One of the reactant must absorb the infra-red CO_2 laser radiation.

The synthesis method is as follows [38]:

- Nanoparticles are produced by this method have been classified as vapor-phase synthesis procedure.
- In the vapor phase when super saturation is reached nanoparticle starts to grow.
- Coalescence and coagulation leads to the growth of the nanoparticle.
- At significant high temperature spherical particles are formed.
- At lower temperature non-spherical or loose agglomerates of particles are formed.

The advantages and disadvantages are as follows in Table **12** [42]:

Table 12. Advantages and disadvantages of Laser pyrolysis method.

Advantages	Disadvantages
Formation of high quality nanoparticles	High temperature is produced
Small sized particles with narrow size distribution	Toxic precursors
Reduced expense	-
Rapid analysis process	-
Absence of contamination	-

Flame Spray Pyrolysis

Sokolowski *et al.* first utilized this method for the synthesis of Al_2O_3 nanoparticle [43]. Later this method is used for oxide and non-oxide ceramic nanoparticle synthesis.

The characteristics of this synthesis method are:

- This method is a one-step combustion process with liquid precursors.
- This procedure contains less volatile precursors, high temperature flames, proven scalability and large temperature gradients.
- This is the most used technique for the fabrication of the nanoparticles.

Nanoparticle fabrication method has several sequential steps as follows [44]:

- Precursors evaporate/decompose forming metal vapors.
- Super saturation leads to the formation of nucleation.
- Growth by coalescence and sintering.
- Particle aggregation and agglomeration.

The advantages and disadvantages are in Table **13** [45 - 47]:

Table 13. Advantages and disadvantages of Flame spray pyrolysis method.

Advantages	Disadvantages
The precursors can be mixed homogeneously	Poor mechanical stability
Only sub sintering temperatures is needed	Precursors are limited to thermally stable materials
High specific surface area of the final product	Safe usage is required
Low cost	-
Controllable particle size	-

Electrospraying

By this method nanoparticles of various morphological structure and types can be synthesized depending upon the solvents used.

The special features of this method are as follows [48]:

- High encapsulation capacity like genes, proteins *etc.*
- Possible to produce solid particles in single step.
- Properties of nanoparticles can be controlled by changing parameters such as

voltage, collector distance, flow rate, viscosity, biopolymer type, density, and concentration of the solvent.

The synthesis method is as follows:

- Mixture of solutions are taken up by the syringe.
- High voltage are produced at the capillary tip for the formation of charged droplets.
- Solvents evaporate and the final product is collected.

The advantages and disadvantages are in Table **14** [49]:

Table 14. Advantages and disadvantages of Electrospraying method.

Advantages	Disadvantages
Controlled shapes and sizes	Delicate engineering
High encapsulation efficiency	Up scaling needs more study
Reduced toxicity	-

Melt Blending

This method is one of the oldest methods of designing polymer composites with NPs as the fillers to achieve desirable material characteristics.

The characteristics of the method are as follows:

- This method is highly environment friendly.
- The procedure is suitable for industrial use.

The synthesis method is as follows:

- For synthesizing nanoparticle the polymer is melted and mixed with the desired amount of the intercalated clay.
- Melting and blending is carried out in the presence of an inert gas, such as argon, nitrogen, or neon.
- Alternatively, the polymer may be mixed with the intercalant and then heated to form the desired clay polymer nanocomposites.

The advantages and disadvantages are in Table **15** [50 - 52]:

Table 15. Advantages and disadvantages of melt blending method.

Advantages	Disadvantages
Environment friendly	Poor dispersion
Potential industrial application	Degradation of the nanoparticle can occur
Cost effective	
Reduced contamination	

BIO-ASSISTED METHODS

The bio-assisted method of nanoparticle synthesis is highly cost effective, low toxic and eco-friendly method. By this method with the help of bacteria, fungus, algae, yeast, nucleic acids, enzymes and plant extracts the nanoparticles are synthesized. This synthesis method is classified into three groups, the first one is when the nanoparticles are synthesized using microorganisms, next is when they are synthesized using macromolecules and lastly when they are synthesized using plant extracts.

Biogenic Synthesis Using Microorganisms

For synthesis of nanoparticles the Prokaryotic bacteria, fungi, actinomycetes, algae and yeast acts as a bio reactor. Varity of nanoparticles are synthesized by this method.

The characteristics of this method are as follows [53]:

- Various application of biogenic synthesis of nanoparticles using bacteria has popularized this method.
- Use of fungi for the synthesis of nanoparticle is highly used method as this system has reception towards toxicity, higher bioaccumulation, cost effective, effortless and simple synthesis method with less biomass handling hazards.
- Yeast mediated synthesis method of nanoparticles is used for huge quantity of nanoparticles extraction.

The synthesis method is as follows:

- Microorganisms targets ions at their environment and by cellular activities it turns the metal ion into elementary metals.
- The synthesis may be intracellular or extracellular depending upon the location where these nanoparticles are synthesized.

- In intracellular method the ions are internalized within the cell and by the help of cellular enzymes they are converted into nanoparticles.
- In the extracellular method the ions are grabbed by the surface of the cell and by extracellular enzymes they are converted into nanoparticles.

The advantages and disadvantages are as follows in Table **16** [54]:

Table 16. Advantages and disadvantages of Biogenic synthesis using microorganisms.

Advantages	Disadvantages
Extracted in ambient temperature	More exploration needed in this area
Low cost	Low performance
Environment friendly	-
Reduced toxicity	-

Biogenic Synthesis Using Bio-molecules as the Templates

In this method of nanoparticle synthesis nucleic acids, membranes, viruses and diatoms are used as templates. In this method virus, proteins and enzymes are also exploited for the synthesis of the same. It was demonstrated how DNA hydrogel could be used and crosslinked before incorporating transition metal ions (*e.g.* gold, Au(III) metal ions) to DNA macromolecules that eventually lead to the formation of Au NPs. This process makes a reduction of Au (III) leading to the formation of Au atoms and metal clusters that develop into Au NPs on the chain of DNA [55].

The characteristics of this method are [56]:

- Various types of DNA with unique sequences can develop specific types of nanoparticles.
- DNA-protein complexes can fabricate various types of nanoparticles.
- Three dimensional structures of RNA molecules can act as a catalyst for the formation of nanoparticles.

The synthesis method is [57]:

- First of all reduction of the ions and formation of cluster of molecules
- Lastly the isolation of the nanoparticles

The advantages and disadvantages are as follows in Table **17**:

Table 17. Advantages and disadvantages of Biogenic synthesis using bio-molecules as the templates.

Advantages	Disadvantages
Low cost	More exploration required
Environment friendly	-

Biogenic Synthesis Using Plant Extracts

Biosynthesis of nanoparticles using plant extract is highly environment friendly method. By this method we can synthesis noble metals, bi-metallic alloys, metal oxides, *etc.* [58].

The characteristics of this method are [53]:

- The gold and silver nanoparticles can be extracted from *Geranium*, *Aloe vera* plant, sundried *Cinnamomum camphora* and *Azadiracta indica* leaf.
- Several other plants can be used for extraction of various types of nanoparticles.

The synthesis method is single step biosynthesis process. Even the capping agent is also supplied by the plant.

The advantages and disadvantages are in the Table **18** [59]:

Table 18. Advantages and disadvantages of Biogenic synthesis using plant extracts.

Advantages	Disadvantages
Very effective	Resources are not always available
Non toxic	All species do not have similar synthesis efficiency
Rapid method	Nonrenewable waste formation
Eco-friendly	Heterogeneous output
Cost effective	Low reproducibility
	Cannot be used for large scale production

CONCLUSION

Since half a century ago, the scientists are continuously exploring new synthesis methods of nanoparticles with optimum size and morphology to use them in divers' field of application (Table **19**). In this study, we are intended to explore the already available synthesis method of nanoparticles that are used in the medicinal field. It is anticipated that this review will help the researchers to find out the suitable synthesis technique to fabricate their desired nanoparticles.

Table 19. Applications of nanoparticles

Nanoparticles	Applications	References
Gold Nanoparticle	Nanomedicines: drug delivery, gene delivery, hyperthermia-assisted cancer phototherapy, photodynamic therapy	[60 - 63]
	Biosensors: highly sensitive optical biosensor, electrochemical biosensor and plasmon resonance biosensors	[64 - 66]
	In-vivo and *ex-vivo* bio-imaging: photon luminescence imaging, magnetic resonance imaging, photo acoustic tomography, Raman imaging, *etc.*	[67]
	Antibacterial activity	[68]
	Solar Cells, Energy Storage application	[69, 70]
Silver Nanoparticle	Nanomedicines: antibacterial applications (textile coating, healthcare, food technology, water disinfection, environmental cleaning,) wound healing, cancer therapeutics	[71 - 74]
	Biosensing: designing highly sensitive biosensor chips/electrodes, biological tagging for quantitative detection	[75, 76]
	Solar cells, electroluminescent displays, optical sensors, surface enhanced Raman spectroscopy, electrical contacts for electrical devices, Catalysis	[77 - 83]
Iron Nanoparticle	Biomedical applications: Biosensors, MRI contrast enhancement, hyperthermia	[84 - 86]
	Magnetic and electrical applications: Magnetic recording media, soft magnetic materials	[87, 88]
	Catalytic applications	[89, 90]
Platinum Nanoparticle	Biomedical applications: affinity probe for the detection of small biomolecules, Catalytic nanomedicines, biosensors	[91 - 93]
	Catalytic applications, Solar Cells	[94, 95]
Palladium Nanoparticle	Surface enhanced Raman scattering and electrocatalysis	[96]
	Catalysis	[97]
	Antibacterial Activity	[98]
	Fuel Cells	[99]
	Biosensors.	[100]
Germanium Nanoparticle	Electronic/Optoelectronic	[101]

(Table 19) cont.....

Nanoparticles	Applications	References
Cerium Oxide	Potential regenerative antioxidant	[102]
	Therapeutic applications for reactive oxygen species (ROS)-related diseases such as Cancer, diabetes, arthritis, infertility, macular degeneration	[103, 104]
	Catalytic convertor for removing toxic gases	[102]
	Solid Oxide fuel cells	[102]
	Biosensors	[105]
	Photocatalysis	[106]
	Antibacterial activity	[107]
Titanium Dioxide	Drug delivery and cellular delivery	[108 - 110]
	Antimicrobial coatings	[111]
	As UV filters in sunscreens, toothpaste, cosmetics, *etc*	[112 - 114]
	Biosensors	[115]
Zinc Oxide	Solar cells	[116]
	Photocatalytic and hygienic coatings Biosensors	[117, 118]
	Important additive for different cosmetics, ointments and food products. Cure activator for rubbers of different kinds	[119]
	Antibacterial	[120]
Ferric Oxide	Development of immunoassays, magnetic resonance imaging contrast agents	[121, 122]
	Targeted drug delivery vehicles, as well as in magnetic hyperthermia.	[123, 124]
Cadmium Sulfide	As fluorescent probes, Optical, electrochemical and photoelectrochemical biosensors	[125 - 127]
	Solar Cells, Photoluminescence devices	[128, 129]
Cadmium Selenide	Solar cells, Light emitting diodes	[130, 131]
Magnetic Nanoparticles	Biomedical applications: Gene delivery, Magnetic resonance imaging, Magnetic carriers for bio-separation	[132 - 134]
	Catalyst supports	[135]
Lanthanides Nanoparticles	*In-Vivo* Cell Imaging	[136]
	Near-infrared photodynamic therapy	[137]
	Light Nano transducers for photo activation applications	[138]

(Table 19) cont.....

Nanoparticles	Applications	References
Carbon Nanoparticles	Cancer diagnostic and therapy	[139, 140]
	Antibacterial	[141]
	Designing of fluorescent imaging probes	[142]
	Catalysis	[32]
	Solar Cells, Protective Coatings and Emission devices	[143 - 145]
Graphene Oxide Nanoparticles	cell delivery In drug delivery for cancer therapeutics Cell therapy	[145 - 149]
	Non-bleaching optical probe for two-photon luminescence Imaging	[149]
	Biosensors	[150]
Polymeric Nanoparticle	Nanomedicines and Drug Delivery	[151 - 153]
	Fluorescent polymeric NPs for cell imaging Photo acoustic Imaging	[154, 155]
	Biosensors	[156]

Appropriate synthesis method identification is important in order to make the final product cost-effective, low toxic and good agent of drug delivery or gene delivery in the cell. This study has broadly discussed the steps involved in the synthesis techniques of nanoparticles with their advantages and drawbacks while using it in the medicinal field.

REFERENCES

[1] Adair JH, Suvaci E. Submicron electroceramic powders by hydrothermal synthesis. In: Buschow KHJ, Cahn RW, Flemings MC, Ilschner B, Kramer EJ, Mahajan S, Eds. Encyclopedia of Materials: Science and Technology. Oxford: Elsevier 2001; pp. 8933-7. [http://dx.doi.org/10.1016/B0-08-043152-6/01607-7]

[2] Dembski S, Schneider C, Christ B, Retter M. 5 - Core-shell nanoparticles and their use for *in vitro* and *in vivo* diagnostics. In: Focarete ML, Tampieri A, Eds. Core-Shell Nanostructures for Drug Delivery and Theranostics. Woodhead Publishing 2018; pp. 119-41. [http://dx.doi.org/10.1016/B978-0-08-102198-9.00005-3]

[3] Athar T. Smart precursors for smart nanoparticles. In: Ahmed W, Jackson MJ, Eds. Emerging Nanotechnologies for Manufacturing. 2nd ed. Boston: William Andrew Publishing 2015; pp. 444-538. [http://dx.doi.org/10.1016/B978-0-323-28990-0.00017-8]

[4] Rane AV, Kanny K, Abitha VK, Thomas S. Methods for synthesis of nanoparticles and fabrication of nanocomposites. In: Mohan Bhagyaraj S, Oluwafemi OS, Kalarikkal N, Thomas S, Eds. Synthesis of Inorganic Nanomaterials. Woodhead Publishing 2018; pp. 121-39. [http://dx.doi.org/10.1016/B978-0-08-101975-7.00005-1]

[5] Cruz IF, Freire C, Araújo JP, Pereira C, Pereira AM. Multifunctional ferrite nanoparticles: from current trends toward the future. In: El-Gendy AA, Barandiarán JM, Hadimani RL, Eds. Magnetic Nanostructured Materials. Elsevier 2018; pp. 59-116. [http://dx.doi.org/10.1016/B978-0-12-813904-2.00003-6]

[6] Baraket L, Ghorbel A. Control preparation of aluminium chromium mixed oxides by Sol-Gel process.

1998.
[http://dx.doi.org/10.1016/S0167-2991(98)80233-4]

[7] Rao BG, Mukherjee D, Reddy BM. Novel approaches for preparation of nanoparticles. Nanostructures for Novel Therapy. Elsevier 2017; pp. 1-36.

[8] Schmidt H. Nanoparticles by chemical synthesis, processing to materials and innovative applications. Appl Organomet Chem 2001; 15: 331-43.
[http://dx.doi.org/10.1002/aoc.169]

[9] Hench LL, West JK. The sol-gel process. Chemical Reviews 1990; 1: 33-72.
[http://dx.doi.org/10.1021/cr00099a003]

[10] Kumar A, Yadav N, Bhatt M, Mishra N, Chaudhary P, Singh R. Sol-Gel derived nanomaterials and it's applications: A review. Res J Chem Sci 2015; 5(12): 1-6.
[http://dx.doi.org/10.3310/hta19670] [PMID: 26307643]

[11] Mitra A, De G. Sol-gel synthesis of metal nanoparticle incorporated oxide films on glass. In: Karmakar B, Rademann K, Stepanov AL, Eds. Glass Nanocomposites. Boston: William Andrew Publishing 2016; pp. 145-63.
[http://dx.doi.org/10.1016/B978-0-323-39309-6.00006-7]

[12] Solanki JN, Murthy ZVP. Controlled size silver nanoparticles synthesis with water-in-oil microemulsion method: A topical review. Industrial & Engineering Chemistry Research 2011; 50(22): 12311-23.
[http://dx.doi.org/10.1021/ie201649x]

[13] Liveri V. Controlled synthesis of nanoparticles in microheterogeneous systems 2006.

[14] Malik MA, Wani MY, Hashim MA. Microemulsion method: A novel route to synthesize organic and inorganic nanomaterials: 1st Nano Update. Arabian J Chemistry. 2012; 5(4): 397-417.

[15] López-Quintela MA, Rivas J, Blanco MC, Tojo C. Synthesis of nanoparticles in microemulsions. In: Liz-Marzán LM, Kamat PV, Eds. Nanoscale Materials Boston, MA. Springer, US 2003; pp. 135-55.

[16] Abedini A, Daud AR, Abdul Hamid MA, Kamil Othman N, Saion E. A review on radiation-induced nucleation and growth of colloidal metallic nanoparticles. Nanoscale Res Lett 2013; 8(1): 474.
[http://dx.doi.org/10.1186/1556-276X-8-474] [PMID: 24225302]

[17] Hayashi H, Hakuta Y. Hydrothermal synthesis of metal oxide nanoparticles in supercritical water. Materials (Basel) 2010; 3(7): 3794-817.
[http://dx.doi.org/10.3390/ma3073794] [PMID: 28883312]

[18] Fiévet F, Ammar-Merah S, Brayner R, *et al.* The polyol process: a unique method for easy access to metal nanoparticles with tailored sizes, shapes and compositions. Chem Soc Rev 2018; 47(14): 5187-233.
[http://dx.doi.org/10.1039/C7CS00777A] [PMID: 29901663]

[19] Rycenga M, Cobley CM, Zeng J, *et al.* Controlling the synthesis and assembly of silver nanostructures for plasmonic applications. Chem Rev 2011; 111(6): 3669-712.
[http://dx.doi.org/10.1021/cr100275d] [PMID: 21395318]

[20] Wiley B, Herricks T, Sun Y, Xia Y. Polyol synthesis of silver nanoparticles: use of chloride and oxygen to promote the formation of single-crystal, truncated cubes and tetrahedrons. Nano Letters 2004; 4(9): 1733-9

[21] Leonard BM, Bhuvanesh NS, Schaak RE. Low-temperature polyol synthesis of $AuCuSn_2$ and $AuNiSn_2$: using solution chemistry to access ternary intermetallic compounds as nanocrystals. J Am Chem Soc 2005; 127(20): 7326-7.
[http://dx.doi.org/10.1021/ja051481v] [PMID: 15898777]

[22] Coskun S, Aksoy B, Unalan H. Polyol synthesis of silver nanowires: an extensive parametric study.

Cryst Growth Des 2011; 09/26(11): 4963-9.
[http://dx.doi.org/10.1021/cg200874g]

[23] Meshesha BT, Barrabés N, Medina F, Sueiras J. Polyol mediated synthesis & characteritzation of Cu nanoparticles: Effect of 1-hexadecylamine as stabilizing agent 2009.

[24] Das RAN. Overview on microwave mediated synthesis. International Journal of Research and Development in Pharmacy and Life Sciences 2012; 06(01)

[25] Gabriel C, Gabriel SH, Grant EH, *et al.* Dielectric parameters relevant to microwave dielectric heating. Chem Soc Rev 1998; 27(3): 213-24.
[http://dx.doi.org/10.1039/a827213z]

[26] Chikan V, McLaurin EJ. Rapid nanoparticle synthesis by magnetic and microwave heating. Nanomaterials (Basel) 2016; 6(5): 85.
[http://dx.doi.org/10.3390/nano6050085] [PMID: 28335212]

[27] Ambrozic G, Orel Z, Zigon M. Microwave-assisted non-aqueous synthesis of ZnO nanoparticles. Materiali in Tehnologije 2011; 45: 173-7.

[28] Makhlouf ASH. Current and advanced coating technologies for industrial applications. In: Makhlouf ASH, Tiginyanu I, Eds. Nanocoatings and Ultra-Thin Films. Woodhead Publishing 2011; pp. 3-23.
[http://dx.doi.org/10.1533/9780857094902.1.3]

[29] O'Brien P. Chemical Vapor Deposition. In: Buschow KHJ, Cahn RW, Flemings MC, Ilschner B, Kramer EJ, Mahajan S, Eds. Encyclopedia of Materials: Science and Technology. Oxford: Elsevier 2001; pp. 1173-6.
[http://dx.doi.org/10.1016/B0-08-043152-6/00219-9]

[30] Yun J, Bae T-S, Kwon J-D, Lee S, Lee G-H. Antireflective silica nanoparticle array directly deposited on flexible polymer substrates by chemical vapor deposition. Nanoscale 2012; 4(22): 7221-30.
[http://dx.doi.org/10.1039/c2nr32381h] [PMID: 23073117]

[31] Hamedani Y, Macha P, Bunning T, Naik R, Vasudev M. Plasma-enhanced chemical vapor deposition: where we are and the outlook for the future. 2016.

[32] Xing T, Sunarso J, Yang W, *et al.* Ball milling: a green mechanochemical approach for synthesis of nitrogen doped carbon nanoparticles. Nanoscale 2013; 5(17): 7970-6.
[http://dx.doi.org/10.1039/c3nr02328a] [PMID: 23864038]

[33] Dhand C, Dwivedi N, Loh XJ, Ng A, Verma N, Beuerman R, *et al.* Methods and strategies for the synthesis of diverse nanoparticles and their applications: a comprehensive overview. RSC Adv 2015 ;5.
[http://dx.doi.org/10.1039/C5RA19388E]

[34] Faraji G, Kim HS, Kashi HT. Introduction. In: Faraji G, Kim HS, Kashi HT, Eds. Severe Plastic Deformation. Elsevier 2018; pp. 1-17.
[http://dx.doi.org/10.1016/B978-0-12-813518-1.00020-5]

[35] Shi D, Guo Z, Bedford N. 5 - Nanomagnetic Materials. In: Shi D, Guo Z, Bedford N, Eds. Nanomaterials and Devices. Oxford: William Andrew Publishing 2015; pp. 105-59.

[36] Birringer R, Gleiter H, Klein HP, Marquardt P. Nanocrystalline materials an approach to a novel solid structure with gas-like disorder? Physics Letters A. 1984 ; 102(8): 365-9.
[http://dx.doi.org/10.1016/0375-9601(84)90300-1]

[37] Kruis FE, Fissan H, Peled A. Synthesis of nanoparticles in the gas phase for electronic, optical and magnetic applications—a review. Journal of Aerosol Science. 1998 ; 29(5): 511-35. 1998.

[38] Wagener P, Barcikowski S, Bärsch N. Fabrication of nanoparticles and nanomaterials using laser ablation in liquids. Photonik international. 2011 : 20-3.

[39] Okuyama K, Wuled Lenggoro I. Preparation of nanoparticles *via* spray route. Chem Eng Sci. 2003 ; 58(3): 537-47.

[http://dx.doi.org/10.1016/S0009-2509(02)00578-X]

[40] Daraio C, Jin S. Synthesis and Patterning Methods for Nanostructures Useful for Biological Applications. 2012; pp. 27-44. [http://dx.doi.org/10.1007/978-0-387-31296-5_2]

[41] D'Amato R, Falconieri M, Gagliardi S, Popovici E, Serra E, Terranova G, *et al.* Synthesis of ceramic nanoparticles by laser pyrolysis: From research to applications. J Anal Appl Pyrolysis 2013; 104: 461-9. 2013.

[42] Sumanth Kumar D, Jai Kumar B, Mahesh HM. Quantum Nanostructures (QDs): An Overview. In: Mohan Bhagyaraj S, Oluwafemi OS, Kalarikkal N, Thomas S, Eds. Synthesis of Inorganic Nanomaterials. Woodhead Publishing 2018; pp. 59-88. [http://dx.doi.org/10.1016/B978-0-08-101975-7.00003-8]

[43] Sokolowski M, Sokolowska A, Michalski A, Gokieli B. The "in-flame-reaction" method for Al_2O_3 aerosol formation. Journal of Aerosol Science 1977; 8(4): 219-30. [http://dx.doi.org/10.1016/0021-8502(77)90041-6]

[44] Choa YH, Yang JK, Kim BH, Jeong YK, Lee JS, Nakayama T, *et al.* Preparation and characterization of metal/ceramic nanoporous nanocomposite powders. J Magn Magn Mater 2003; 266(1): 12-9.

[45] Nunes D, Pimentel A, Santos L, Barquinha P, Pereira L, Fortunato E, *et al.* Synthesis, design, and morphology of metal oxide nanostructures. In: Nunes D, Pimentel A, Santos L, Barquinha P, Pereira L, Fortunato E, Eds. Metal Oxide Nanostructures. Elsevier 2019; pp. 21-57. [http://dx.doi.org/10.1016/B978-0-12-811512-1.00002-3]

[46] Lee J-H. 4 - Technological realization of semiconducting metal oxide–based gas sensors. In: Barsan N, Schierbaum K, Eds. Gas Sensors Based on Conducting Metal Oxides. Elsevier 2019; pp. 167-216. [http://dx.doi.org/10.1016/B978-0-12-811224-3.00004-4]

[47] Virji MA, Stefaniak AB. 8.06 - A Review of Engineered Nanomaterial Manufacturing Processes and Associated Exposures. In: Hashmi S, Batalha GF, Van Tyne CJ, Yilbas B, Eds. Comprehensive Materials Processing. Oxford: Elsevier 2014; pp. 103-25. [http://dx.doi.org/10.1016/B978-0-08-096532-1.00811-6]

[48] Jafari SM, McClements DJ. Chapter One - Nanotechnology Approaches for Increasing Nutrient Bioavailability. In: Toldrá F, Ed. Advances in Food and Nutrition Research 81. Academic Press 2017; pp. 1-30.

[49] Wang J, Jansen JA, Yang F. Electrospraying: possibilities and challenges of engineering carriers for biomedical applications—a mini review. Frontiers in Chemistry 2019; 7(258).

[50] Verma D, Goh KL. Chapter 11 - Functionalized Graphene-Based Nanocomposites for Energy Applications. In: Jawaid M, Bouhfid R, Kacem Qaiss Ae, editors. Functionalized Graphene Nanocomposites and their Derivatives: Elsevier; 2019. p. 219-43. 2019.

[51] Vasudeo Rane A, Kanny K, Abitha VK, Patil SS, Thomas S. Clay–Polymer Composites: Design of Clay Polymer Nanocomposite by Mixing. In: Jlassi K, Chehimi MM, Thomas S, Eds. Clay-Polymer Nanocomposites. Elsevier 2017; pp. 113-44. [http://dx.doi.org/10.1016/B978-0-323-46153-5.00004-5]

[52] Lin B, Sundararaj U, Pötschke P. Melt mixing of polycarbonate with multi-walled carbon nanotubes in miniature mixers. Macromol Mater Eng 2006; 03/14(291): 227-38. [http://dx.doi.org/10.1002/mame.200500335]

[53] Chaudhari A. Biogenic Synthesis of Nanoparticles and Potential Applications An Eco-friendly Approach. J Nanomed Nanotechnol 2013; 4: 165.

[54] Parveen K, Banse V, Ledwani L. Green synthesis of nanoparticles: Their advantages and disadvantages. AIP Conference Proceedings. 2016; 1724(1): 020048. 1724.

[55] Zinchenko A, Miwa Y, Lopatina LI, Sergeyev VG, Murata S. DNA hydrogel as a template for

synthesis of ultrasmall gold nanoparticles for catalytic applications. ACS applied materials & interfaces. 2014; 6(5): 3226-32.
[http://dx.doi.org/10.1021/am5008886]

[56] Zhou L, Ren J, Qu X. Nucleic acid-templated functional nanocomposites for biomedical applications. Materials Today. 2017; 20(4): 179-90.
[http://dx.doi.org/10.1016/j.mattod.2016.09.012]

[57] Willner I, Willner B. Biomolecule-based nanomaterials and nanostructures. Nano Lett 2010; 10(10). 3805-15.
[http://dx.doi.org/10.1021/nl102083j] [PMID: 20843088]

[58] Iravani S. Green synthesis of metal nanoparticles using plants. Green Chem 2011; 13(10): 2638-50.
[http://dx.doi.org/10.1039/c1gc15386b]

[59] Das M, Chatterjee S. Chapter 11 - Green synthesis of metal/metal oxide nanoparticles toward biomedical applications: Boon or bane. In: Shukla AK, Iravani S, editors. Green Synthesis, Characterization and Applications of Nanoparticles: Elsevier; 2019. p. 265-301.

[60] Khan A, Rashid R, Murtaza G, Zahra A. Gold nanoparticles: Synthesis and applications in drug delivery. Tropical Journal of Pharmaceutical Research. 2014; 13: 1169-77. 2014.

[61] Chatterjee DK, Diagaradjane P, Krishnan S. Nanoparticle-mediated hyperthermia in cancer therapy. Ther Deliv 2011; 2(8): 1001-14.
[http://dx.doi.org/10.4155/tde.11.72] [PMID: 22506095]

[62] Ye E, Regulacio MD, Zhang S-Y, Loh XJ, Han M-Y. Anisotropically branched metal nanostructures. Chem Soc Rev 2015; 44(17): 6001-17.
[http://dx.doi.org/10.1039/C5CS00213C] [PMID: 26065370]

[63] Oo MK, Yang X, Du H, Wang H. 5-aminolevulinic acid-conjugated gold nanoparticles for photodynamic therapy of cancer. Nanomed (Lond) 2008; 3(6): 777-86.
[http://dx.doi.org/10.2217/17435889.3.6.777] [PMID: 19025452]

[64] Pandey P, Singh SP, Arya SK, *et al.* Application of thiolated gold nanoparticles for the enhancement of glucose oxidase activity. Langmuir 2007; 23(6): 3333-7.
[http://dx.doi.org/10.1021/la062901c] [PMID: 17261046]

[65] Pingarrón JM, Yáñez-Sedeño P, González-Cortés A. Gold nanoparticle-based electrochemical biosensors. Electrochimica Acta 2008; 53(19): 5848-66.
[http://dx.doi.org/10.1016/j.electacta.2008.03.005]

[66] Lee J-H, Cho H-Y, Choi HK, Lee J-Y, Choi J-W. Application of gold nanoparticle to plasmonic biosensors. Int J Mol Sci 2018; 19(7): 2021.
[http://dx.doi.org/10.3390/ijms19072021] [PMID: 29997363]

[67] Cai W, Gao T, Hong H, Sun J. Applications of gold nanoparticles in cancer nanotechnology. Nanotechnol Sci Appl 2008; 1: 17-32.
[http://dx.doi.org/10.2147/NSA.S3788] [PMID: 24198458]

[68] Lima E, Guerra R, Lara V, Guzmán A. Gold nanoparticles as efficient antimicrobial agents for Escherichia coli and Salmonella typhi. Chem Cent J. 2013; 7(1): 11
[http://dx.doi.org/10.1186/1752-153X-7-11]

[69] Wang C, Choy W, Duan C, Fung D, Sha W, Xie F, *et al.* Optical and electrical effects of gold nanoparticles in the active layer of polymer solar cells. J Mater Chem 2011; 12/13(22): 1206-11.

[70] Anjana PM, Bindhu MR, Rakhi RB. Green synthesized gold nanoparticle dispersed porous carbon composites for electrochemical energy storage. Mater Sci Technol 2019; 2(3): 389-95. ;
[http://dx.doi.org/10.1016/j.mset.2019.03.006]

[71] Abou El-Nour KMM, Eftaiha Aa, Al-Warthan A, Ammar RAA. Synthesis and applications of silver nanoparticles. Arab. J. Chem 2010; 3(3): 135-40.

[http://dx.doi.org/10.1016/j.arabjc.2010.04.008]

[72] Rigo C, Ferroni L, Tocco I, *et al.* Active silver nanoparticles for wound healing. Int J Mol Sci 2013; 14(3): 4817-40.
[http://dx.doi.org/10.3390/ijms14034817] [PMID: 23455461]

[73] Ambrogi V, Donnadio A, Pietrella D, *et al.* Chitosan films containing mesoporous SBA-15 supported silver nanoparticles for wound dressing. J Mater Chem B Mater Biol Med 2014; 2(36): 6054-63.
[http://dx.doi.org/10.1039/C4TB00927D] [PMID: 32261857]

[74] Jeyaraj M, Sathishkumar G, Sivanandhan G, *et al.* Biogenic silver nanoparticles for cancer treatment: an experimental report. Colloids Surf B Biointerfaces 2013; 106: 86-92.
[http://dx.doi.org/10.1016/j.colsurfb.2013.01.027] [PMID: 23434696]

[75] Fan M, Thompson M, Andrade ML, Brolo AG. Silver nanoparticles on a plastic platform for localized surface plasmon resonance biosensing. Anal Chem 2010; 82(15): 6350-2.
[http://dx.doi.org/10.1021/ac101495m]

[76] Mukherjee S, Chowdhury D, Kotcherlakota R, *et al.* Potential theranostics application of bio-synthesized silver nanoparticles (4-in-1 system). Theranostics 2014; 4(3): 316-35.
[http://dx.doi.org/10.7150/thno.7819] [PMID: 24505239]

[77] Park J-W, Ullah M, Park S, Ha C-S. Organic electroluminescent devices using quantum-size silver nanoparticles. J Mater Sci Mater Electron 2007; 18(1): 393-7.
[http://dx.doi.org/10.1007/s10854-007-9232-6]

[78] Stamplecoskie KG, Scaiano JC, Tiwari VS, Anis H. Optimal size of silver nanoparticles for surface-enhanced raman spectroscopy. J Phys Chem 2011; 115(5): 1403-9.
[http://dx.doi.org/10.1021/jp106666t]

[79] Santos KdO, Elias WC, Signori AM, Giacomelli FC, Yang H, Domingos JB. Synthesis and catalytic properties of silver nanoparticle–linear polyethylene imine colloidal systems. J Phys Chem 2012; 116(7): 4594-604.

[80] Liu P, Liu J, Cheng S, Cai W, Yu F, Zhang Y, *et al.* A high-performance electrode for supercapacitors: Silver nanoparticles grown on a porous perovskite-type material La0.7Sr0.3CoO3−δ substrate. Chem Eng J 2017; 328: 1-10.

[81] Majumdar D, Singha A, Mondal PK, Kundu S. DNA-mediated wirelike clusters of silver nanoparticles: an ultrasensitive SERS substrate. ACS Appl Mater Interfaces 2013; 5(16): 7798-807.
[http://dx.doi.org/10.1021/am402448j] [PMID: 23895297]

[82] Kundu S. Formation of self-assembled Ag nanoparticles on DNA chains with enhanced catalytic activity. Phys Chem Chem Phys 2013; 15(33): 14107-19.
[http://dx.doi.org/10.1039/c3cp51890f] [PMID: 23872921]

[83] D'Andrea C, Neri F, Ossi PM, Santo N, Trusso S. The controlled pulsed laser deposition of Ag nanoparticle arrays for surface enhanced Raman scattering. Nanotechnology 2009; 20(24): 245606.
[http://dx.doi.org/10.1088/0957-4484/20/24/245606] [PMID: 19471080]

[84] Sharma R, Agrawal VV, Srivastava AK, *et al.* Phase control of nanostructured iron oxide for application to biosensor. J Mater Chem B Mater Biol Med 2013; 1(4): 464-74.
[http://dx.doi.org/10.1039/C2TB00192F] [PMID: 32260817]

[85] Lee N, Hyeon T. Designed synthesis of uniformly sized iron oxide nanoparticles for efficient magnetic resonance imaging contrast agents. Chem Soc Rev 2012; 41(7): 2575-89.
[http://dx.doi.org/10.1039/C1CS15248C] [PMID: 22138852]

[86] Huber DL. Synthesis, properties, and applications of iron nanoparticles. Small 2005; 1(5): 482-501.
[http://dx.doi.org/10.1002/smll.200500006] [PMID: 17193474]

[87] Singamaneni S, Bliznyuk VN, Binek C, Tsymbal EY. Magnetic nanoparticles: recent advances in synthesis, self-assembly and applications. J Mater Chem 2011; 21(42): 16819-45.

[http://dx.doi.org/10.1039/c1jm11845e]

[88] Bao Y, Wen T, Samia ACS, Khandhar A, Krishnan KM. Magnetic nanoparticles: material engineering and emerging applications in lithography and biomedicine. J Mater Sci. 2016; 51(1): 513-53. PubMed PMID: 26586919. Epub 09/01. eng.

[89] Lopez-Tejedor D, Benavente R, Palomo JM. Iron nanostructured catalysts: design and applications. Catal Sci Technol 2018; 8(7): 1754-76. [http://dx.doi.org/10.1039/C7CY02259J]

[90] Parimala L, Santhanalakshmi J. Studies on the iron nanoparticles catalyzed reduction of substituted aromatic ketones to alcohols. J Nanoparticles. 2014; 156868. [http://dx.doi.org/10.1155/2014/156868]

[91] Shrivas K, Agrawal K, Wu H-F. Application of platinum nanoparticles as affinity probe and matrix for direct analysis of small biomolecules and microwave digested proteins using matrix-assisted laser desorption/ionization mass spectrometry. Analyst 2011; 136(13): 2852-7. 2011.

[92] López T, Figueras F, Manjarrez J, Bustos J, Alvarez M, Silvestre-Albero J, *et al.* Catalytic nanomedicine: A new field in antitumor treatment using supported platinum nanoparticles. *In vitro* DNA degradation and *in vivo* tests with C6 animal model on Wistar rats. Eur J Med Chem 2010; 45(5): 1982-90.

[93] Claussen JC, Kumar A, Jaroch DB, Khawaja MH, Hibbard AB, Porterfield DM, *et al.* Biosensors: nanostructuring platinum nanoparticles on multilayered graphene petal nanosheets for electrochemical biosensing. Adv Funct Mater 2012; 22(16): 3317. [http://dx.doi.org/10.1002/adfm.201290096]

[94] Mostafa S, Behafarid F, Croy JR, Ono LK, Li L, Yang JC, *et al.* Shape-dependent catalytic properties of pt nanoparticles. J Am Chem Soc 2010; 132(44): 15714-9 [http://dx.doi.org/10.1021/ja106679z]

[95] Peng KQ, Wang X, Wu XL, Lee ST. Platinum nanoparticle decorated silicon nanowires for efficient solar energy conversion. Nano Lett 2009; 9(11): 3704-9. [http://dx.doi.org/10.1021/nl901734e] [PMID: 19807069]

[96] Chen H, Wei G, Ispas A, Hickey SG, Eychmüller A. Synthesis of palladium nanoparticles and their applications for surface-enhanced raman scattering and electrocatalysis. J. Phys. Chem 2010; 114 (50): 21976-81. [http://dx.doi.org/10.1021/jp106623y]

[97] Xu L, Wu X-C, Zhu J-J. Green preparation and catalytic application of Pd nanoparticles. Nanotechnology. 2008; 19: 305603. [http://dx.doi.org/10.1088/0957-4484/19/30/305603]

[98] Adams CP, Walker KA, Obare SO, Docherty KM. Size-dependent antimicrobial effects of novel palladium nanoparticles. PLoS One. 2014; 9(1): e85981-e. [PMID: 24465824]

[99] Ko Y-J, Kim J-Y, Lee K-S, Park J-K, Baik Y-J, Choi H-J, *et al.* Palladium nanoparticles from surfactant/fast-reduction combination one-pot synthesis for the liquid fuel cell applications. International Journal of Hydrogen Energy. 2018; 43(41): 19029-37.

[100] Lim SH, Wei J, Lin J, Li Q, KuaYou J. A glucose biosensor based on electrodeposition of palladium nanoparticles and glucose oxidase onto Nafion-solubilized carbon nanotube electrode. Biosens Bioelectron 2005; 20(11): 2341-6.

[101] Ichida D, Uchida G, Seo H, Kamataki K, Itagaki N, Koga K, *et al.* Deposition of crystalline Ge nanoparticle films by high-pressure RF magnetron sputtering method. Journal of Physics: Conference Series. 2014; 518: 012002. [http://dx.doi.org/10.1088/1742-6596/518/1/012002]

[102] Das S, Dowding JM, Klump KE, McGinnis JF, Self W, Seal S. Cerium oxide nanoparticles:

applications and prospects in nanomedicine. Nanomedicine (Lond) 2013; 8(9): 1483-508. [http://dx.doi.org/10.2217/nnm.13.133] [PMID: 23987111]

[103] Gao Y, Chen K, Ma J-L, Gao F. Cerium oxide nanoparticles in cancer 2014. http://europepmc.org/abstract/MED/24920925
[http://dx.doi.org/10.2147/OTT.S62057]

[104] Wason MS, Zhao J. Cerium oxide nanoparticles: potential applications for cancer and other diseases. Am J Transl Res 2013; 5(2): 126-31.
[PMID: 23573358]

[105] Charbgoo F, Ramezani M, Darroudi M. Bio-sensing applications of cerium oxide nanoparticles: Advantages and disadvantages. Biosens Bioelectron 2017; 96: 33-43.
[http://dx.doi.org/10.1016/j.bios.2017.04.037] [PMID: 28458132]

[106] Channei D, Inceesungvorn B, Wetchakun N, Phanichphant S, Nakaruk A, Koshy P, *et al.* Photocatalytic activity under visible light of Fe-doped CeO_2 nanoparticles synthesized by flame spray pyrolysis. Ceramics International 2013; 39: 3129-34.

[107] Shah V, Shah S, Shah H, *et al.* Antibacterial activity of polymer coated cerium oxide nanoparticles. PLoS One 2012; 7(10): e47827.
[http://dx.doi.org/10.1371/journal.pone.0047827] [PMID: 23110109]

[108] Hasanzadeh Kafshgari M, Goldmann WH. Insights into theranostic properties of titanium dioxide for nanomedicine. Nano-Micro Letters 2020; 12(1): 22.
[http://dx.doi.org/10.1007/s40820-019-0362-1]

[109] Devanand Venkatasubbu G, Ramasamy S, Ramakrishnan V, Kumar J. Folate targeted PEGylated titanium dioxide nanoparticles as a nanocarrier for targeted paclitaxel drug delivery. Advanced Powder Technology 2013; 24(6): 947-54.
[http://dx.doi.org/10.1016/j.apt.2013.01.008]

[110] Jana B, Mondal G, Biswas A, Chakraborty I, Ghosh S. Functionalised TiO_2 nanoparticles deliver oligo-histidine and avidin tagged biomolecules simultaneously into the cell. RSC Adv 2013; 3(22): 8215-9.
[http://dx.doi.org/10.1039/c3ra41068d]

[111] Prachi P. Antimicrobial titanium dioxide coatings activated by indoor light. C&EN Global Enterprise. 2019; 97(8): 7.

[112] Smijs TG, Pavel S. Titanium dioxide and zinc oxide nanoparticles in sunscreens: focus on their safety and effectiveness. Nanotechnol Sci Appl 2011; 4: 95-112.
[http://dx.doi.org/10.2147/NSA.S19419] [PMID: 24198489]

[113] Rompelberg C, Heringa MB, van Donkersgoed G, *et al.* Oral intake of added titanium dioxide and its nanofraction from food products, food supplements and toothpaste by the Dutch population. Nanotoxicology 2016; 10(10): 1404-14.
[http://dx.doi.org/10.1080/17435390.2016.1222457] [PMID: 27619007]

[114] Dréno B, Alexis A, Chuberre B, Marinovich M. Safety of titanium dioxide nanoparticles in cosmetics. J Eur Acad Dermatol Venereol 2019; 33 (Suppl. 7): 34-46.
[http://dx.doi.org/10.1111/jdv.15943] [PMID: 31588611]

[115] Casero E, Alonso C, Petit-Domínguez MD, Vázquez L, Parra-Alfambra AM, Merino P, *et al.* Lactate biosensor based on a bionanocomposite composed of titanium oxide nanoparticles, photocatalytically reduced graphene, and lactate oxidase. Microchimica Acta. 2014; 181(1): 79-87.
[http://dx.doi.org/10.1007/s00604-013-1070-z]

[116] Ibrahem MA, Wei H-Y, Tsai M-H, Ho K-C, Shyue J-J, Chu CW. Solution-processed zinc oxide nanoparticles as interlayer materials for inverted organic solar cells. Solar Energy Materials and Solar Cells. 2013; 108: 156-63.
[http://dx.doi.org/10.1016/j.solmat.2012.09.007]

[117] Ren X, Chen D, Meng X, Tang F, Hou X, Han D, *et al.* Zinc oxide nanoparticles/glucose oxidase photoelectrochemical system for the fabrication of biosensor. J Colloid Interface Sci. 2009; 334(2): 183-7. PMID: 19394953.

[118] Jašková V, Hochmannová L, Vytřasová J. Nanoparticles in photocatalytic and hygienic coatings. International Journal of Photoenergy. 2013; 2013: 795060. 2013.

[119] Sahoo S, Maiti M, Ganguly A, Jacob George J, Bhowmick AK. Effect of zinc oxide nanoparticles as cure activator on the properties of natural rubber and nitrile rubber. J Appl Polym Sci 2007; 105(4): 2407-15.
[http://dx.doi.org/10.1002/app.26296]

[120] Salah N, Habib SS, Khan ZH, *et al.* High-energy ball milling technique for ZnO nanoparticles as antibacterial material. Int J Nanomedicine 2011; 6: 863-9.
[http://dx.doi.org/10.2147/IJN.S18267] [PMID: 21720499]

[121] Teja AS, Koh P-Y. Synthesis, properties, and applications of magnetic iron oxide nanoparticles. Progress in Crystal Growth and Characterization of Materials. 2009; 55(1): 22-45.
[http://dx.doi.org/10.1016/j.pcrysgrow.2008.08.003]

[122] Marashdeh MW, Ababneh B, Lemine OM, Alsadig A, Omri K, El Mir L, *et al.* The significant effect of size and concentrations of iron oxide nanoparticles on magnetic resonance imaging contrast enhancement. Results in Physics. 2019; 15: 102651.
[http://dx.doi.org/10.1016/j.rinp.2019.102651]

[123] Peng H, Huang Q, Wu T, Wen J, He H. Preparation of Porous γ-Fe2O3@mWO3 Multifunctional Nanoparticles for Drug Loading and Controlled Release. Curr Drug Deliv 2018; 15(2): 278-85.
[http://dx.doi.org/10.2174/1567201814666170224144217] [PMID: 28240176]

[124] Lemine OM, Omri K, Lassaad EM, Velasco V, Crespo P, de la Presa P, *et al.* Fe_2O_3 nanoparticles for magnetic hyperthermia applications. MRS Proceedings. 1779.

[125] Wang L-Y, Wang L, Gao F, Yu Z-Y, Wu Z-M. Application of functionalized CdS nanoparticles as fluorescence probe in the determination of nucleic acids. Analyst. 2002; 127: 977-80.
[http://dx.doi.org/10.1039/b200253c]

[126] Tang J, Wang Y, Li J, Da P, Geng J, Zheng G. Sensitive enzymatic glucose detection by TiO2 nanowire photoelectrochemical biosensors. J Mater Chem A Mater Energy Sustain 2014; 2(17): 6153-7.
[http://dx.doi.org/10.1039/C3TA14173J]

[127] Meissner D, Memming R, Kastening B. Photoelectrochemistry of cadmium sulfide. 1. Reanalysis of photocorrosion and flat-band potential. J. Phys Chem A 1988; 92(12): 3476-83. 1988.

[128] Cortina-Marrero H, Martinez C, Castillo-Ortega M, Hu H. Cellulose acetate fibers covered by CdS nanoparticles for hybrid solar cell applications. Mater Sci Eng B 2012; 09/20(177): 1491-6.
[http://dx.doi.org/10.1016/j.mseb.2012.02.014]

[129] Suhail AM, Khalifa MJ, Saeed NM, Ibrahim OA. White light generation from CdS nanoparticles illuminated by UV-LED. Eur Phy J App Phy 2020; 49(3): 30601.

[130] Lokteva I, Radychev N, Witt F, Borchert H, Parisi J, Kolny-Olesiak J. Surface treatment of cdse nanoparticles for application in hybrid solar cells: the effect of multiple ligand exchange with pyridine. J Phys Chem C 2010; 06/30(114): 12784-91.
[http://dx.doi.org/10.1021/jp103300v]

[131] Schreuder MA, Xiao K, Ivanov IN, Weiss SM, Rosenthal SJ. White light-emitting diodes based on ultrasmall CdSe nanocrystal electroluminescence. Nano Lett 2010; 10(2): 573-6.
[http://dx.doi.org/10.1021/nl903515g] [PMID: 20063863]

[132] Loh XJ, Lee T-C, Dou Q, Deen GR. Utilising inorganic nanocarriers for gene delivery. Biomater Sci 2016; 4(1): 70-86.

[http://dx.doi.org/10.1039/C5BM00277J] [PMID: 26484365]

[133] Perez JM, Josephson L, O'Loughlin T, Högemann D, Weissleder R. Magnetic relaxation switches capable of sensing molecular interactions. Nat Biotechnol 2002; 20(8): 816-20. [http://dx.doi.org/10.1038/nbt720] [PMID: 12134166]

[134] Doyle PS, Bibette J, Bancaud A, Viovy J-L. Self-assembled magnetic matrices for DNA separation chips. Science 2002; 295(5563): 2237. [http://dx.doi.org/10.1126/science.1068420] [PMID: 11910102]

[135] Yoon T-J, Lee W, Oh Y-S, Lee J-K. Magnetic nanoparticles as a catalyst vehicle for simple and easy recycling. New J Chem 2003; 27(2): 227-9. [http://dx.doi.org/10.1039/b209391j]

[136] Wong HT, Tsang MK, Chan CF, Wong KL, Fei B, Hao J. *In vitro* cell imaging using multifunctional small sized KGdF4:Yb3+,Er3+ upconverting nanoparticles synthesized by a one-pot solvothermal process. Nanoscale 2013; 5(8): 3465-73. [http://dx.doi.org/10.1039/c3nr00081h] [PMID: 23475279]

[137] Dou QQ, Teng CP, Ye E, Loh XJ. Effective near-infrared photodynamic therapy assisted by upconversion nanoparticles conjugated with photosensitizers. Int J Nanomedicine 2015; 10: 419-32. [PMID: 25609954]

[138] Idris NM, Jayakumar MKG, Bansal A, Zhang Y. Upconversion nanoparticles as versatile light nanotransducers for photoactivation applications. Chem Soc Rev 2015; 44(6): 1449-78. [http://dx.doi.org/10.1039/C4CS00158C] [PMID: 24969662]

[139] Rani R, Kumar V, Rizzolio F. Fluorescent Carbon Nanoparticles in Medicine for Cancer Therapy: An Update. ACS Med Chem Lett 2017; 9(1): 4-5. [http://dx.doi.org/10.1021/acsmedchemlett.7b00523] [PMID: 29348802]

[140] Tu X, Ma Y, Cao Y, Huang J, Zhang M, Zhang Z. PEGylated carbon nanoparticles for efficient *in vitro* photothermal cancer therapy. J Mater Chem B Mater Biol Med 2014; 2(15): 2184-92. [http://dx.doi.org/10.1039/C3TB21750G] [PMID: 32261502]

[141] Dou Q, Fang X, Jiang S, Chee PL, Lee T-C, Loh XJ. Multi-functional fluorescent carbon dots with antibacterial and gene delivery properties. RSC Advances 2015; 5(58): 46817-22. [http://dx.doi.org/10.1039/C5RA07968C]

[142] Bhunia SK, Saha A, Maity AR, Ray SC, Jana NR. Carbon nanoparticle-based fluorescent bioimaging probes. Sci Rep 2013; 3(1): 1473. [http://dx.doi.org/10.1038/srep01473]

[143] Dwivedi N, Kumar S, Malik HK. Nanostructured titanium/diamond-like carbon multilayer films: deposition, characterization, and applications. ACS applied materials & interfaces. 2011; 3(11): 4268-78.

[144] Dwivedi N, Kumar S, Tripathi RK, Malik HK, Panwar OS. Field emission, morphological and mechanical properties of variety of diamond-like carbon thin films. Applied Physics A. 2011; 105(2):417-25. [http://dx.doi.org/10.1007/s00339-011-6556-0]

[145] Zhu Y, Murali S, Cai W, Li X, Suk JW, Potts JR, *et al.* Graphene and graphene oxide: synthesis, properties, and applications. Advanced materials (Deerfield Beach, Fla) 2010; 22(35): 3906-24. [PMID: 20706983]

[146] Jana B, Biswas A, Mohapatra S, Saha A, Ghosh S. Single functionalized graphene oxide reconstitutes kinesin mediated intracellular cargo transport and delivers multiple cytoskeleton proteins and therapeutic molecules into the cell. Chem Comm (Cambridge, England). 2014; 50(78): 11595-8. [http://dx.doi.org/10.1039/C4CC04924A]

[147] Jana B, Mondal G, Biswas A, *et al.* Dual functionalized graphene oxide serves as a carrier for delivering oligohistidine- and biotin-tagged biomolecules into cells. Macromol Biosci 2013; 13(11):

1478-84.
[http://dx.doi.org/10.1002/mabi.201300129] [PMID: 23894114]

[148] Zhao X, Yang L, Li X, *et al.* Functionalized graphene oxide nanoparticles for cancer cell-specific delivery of antitumor drug. Bioconjug Chem 2015; 26(1): 128-36.
[http://dx.doi.org/10.1021/bc5005137] [PMID: 25525819]

[149] Li JL, Bao HC, Hou XL, Sun L, Wang XG, Gu M. Graphene oxide nanoparticles as a nonbleaching optical probe for two-photon luminescence imaging and cell therapy. Angew Chem Int Ed Engl 2012; 51(8): 1830-4.
[http://dx.doi.org/10.1002/anie.201106102] [PMID: 22247035]

[150] Mukherjee MD, Dhand C, Dwivedi N, Singh BP, Sumana G, Agarwal VV, *et al.* Facile synthesis of 2-dimensional transparent graphene flakes for nucleic acid detection. Sens. Actuators, B 2015; 210: 281-9.

[151] Crucho CI. Stimuli-responsive polymeric nanoparticles for nanomedicine. ChemMedChem 2015; 10(1): 24-38.
[http://dx.doi.org/10.1002/cmdc.201402290] [PMID: 25319803]

[152] Dhand C, Prabhakaran MP, Beuerman RW, Lakshminarayanan R, Dwivedi N, Ramakrishna S. Role of size of drug delivery carriers for pulmonary and intravenous administration with emphasis on cancer therapeutics and lung-targeted drug delivery. RSC Advances 2014; 4(62): 32673-89.
[http://dx.doi.org/10.1039/C4RA02861A]

[153] Elsabahy M, Wooley KL. Design of polymeric nanoparticles for biomedical delivery applications. Chem Soc Rev 2012; 41(7): 2545-61.
[http://dx.doi.org/10.1039/c2cs15327k] [PMID: 22334259]

[154] Li K, Liu B. Polymer-encapsulated organic nanoparticles for fluorescence and photoacoustic imaging. Chem Soc Rev 2014; 43(18): 6570-97.
[http://dx.doi.org/10.1039/C4CS00014E] [PMID: 24792930]

[155] Wang K, Zhang X, Zhang X, Yang B, Li Z, Zhang Q, *et al.* Fabrication of cross-linked fluorescent polymer nanoparticles and their cell imaging applications. J Mater Chem C 2015; 3(8): 1854-60.
[http://dx.doi.org/10.1039/C4TC02672A]

[156] Dhand C, Mukherjee M, Sumana G, Srivastava A, Pandey M, Kim C, *et al.* Preparation, characterization and application of polyaniline nanospheres to biosensing. Nanoscale 2010; 2: 747-54.
[http://dx.doi.org/10.1039/b9nr00346k]

CHAPTER 3

Recent Progress of Nanoparticles Used in the Diagnosis of Different Types of Diseases

Abstract: Nanoparticles used in the detection of biomolecules are being possibly used due to their physical and chemical properties that optimize them with unique characteristics. These properties enable the diagnosis of several disease conditions to make them available for treatment. This study is intended to discuss the emergence of this area and help the researchers in further progress in this field.

This study discusses the disadvantages of the use of currently available methods for diagnostic purposes. It also examines the advantages of the use of nanoparticles in this field of study. This study reviews the properties of metallic nanoparticles including gold and silver, and also quantum dot, silica nanoparticles, *etc.*

Nanotechnology has extended the limitation of the current diagnostic procedures. The potential of using nanoparticles in the diagnosis of diseases is unlimited. Safety study is needed for *in vivo* uses. Nanobiotechnology in clinical uses will play a valuable role in the future development of nanomedicines also.

Keywords: Colorimetric detection, Electrochemical-based detection, ELISA, Emission-based detection, FLISA, Fluorescence based detection, FRET, Gold nanoparticle, Magnetic-based detection, MEF, Microarray detection, MRI, NMR, Plasmonics-based detection, Quantum dot, Quenching, SEIRF, SERS, Silica nanoparticle, Silver nanoparticle.

INTRODUCTION

Currently, the diagnostic tests that are available in the market are mainly based on PCR (polymerase chain reaction) and ELISA (Enzyme-linked Immunosorbant assay). But these diagnostic tests have several drawbacks such as they are time-consuming, expensive, complex and varied accuracy [1]. These issues need to be addressed in the current research scenario. Nanoparticles have several advantages as well as several drawbacks while addressing these problems of the diagnostics used in today's world.

The nanoparticles are not larger than 100nm in size. As the size decreases, their many physical and chemical properties give rise to optical and magnetic

Rituparna Acharya

properties that make them unique for the diagnostic purpose *in vivo*. Molecular diagnosis using nanoparticles is the essential part for the development of personalized medicines. Nano probes help in the diagnosis at the molecular level from cell to organelles. They can be used to improve PCR and non-PCR methods of medical diagnostics. The use of nanoparticles is advantageous as while performing the test, they are needed in a very small amount. They are highly sensitive and by using these materials, the tagging and labeling are faster.

The rapid evolution of nanotechnology has overcome the above-mentioned disadvantages of organic dye and changed the bioanalytical measurement landscape. Several nanoparticles such as gold, silver, quantum dot, and metallic nanoparticles have been developed that have highly sensitive and high specificity for the detection of biomolecules. Minute bioengineering has made these particles small, stable, readily biofunctionalized and easily detectable *in vivo* [2].

In this study, we are intended to find out the major diagnostic ways that can be utilized using nanoparticles. Moreover, we have highlighted the key fundamental properties of the nanoparticles that make them unique for the diagnostic application.

NANOPARTICLE BASED DIAGNOSIS

The research of nanoparticles for diagnostic purposes is facing several challenges. One challenge out of many is the optimization of a nanoparticle for biosensors and the next is the characterization of nanoparticles to make them an ideal diagnostic tool. The problem of development of an optimum nanoparticle is amplified when we face more hurdles such as, we need to develop a nanoparticle that will remain in the suspension for a longer period of time, moreover, there is difficulty in the maintenance of stoichiometry of the reaction between the analyte and the nanoparticle and the problem of cross-reactivity and nonspecific absorption.

However, before addressing the above challenges, the next section deals with nanoparticle based detection methods such as 1) Emission-based Detection, 2) Magnetic-based Detection, 3) Electrochemical-based Detection and lastly, 4) Plasmonics-based Detection.

Emission-Based Detection

Emission-based detection is a two-phase method where the nanoparticle is excited by photon and the emission is recorded. There are several alternative methods such as the use of organic dye but they have drawbacks *i.e.*, they undergo faster photobleaching. On the other hand, when nanoparticles are used, they have several advantages, such as nanoparticles can be manipulated in their excitation and emission wavelengths, and photobleaching does not affect them. Emission-based detection can be of several forms such as fluorescence-based, colorimetric, *etc.*

Fluorescence-Based Detection

Fluorescence-based detection method is a commonly used method for biosensing as it is a simple and highly sensitive method of detection. Today in this era of nanotechnology and nanoparticles, the traditional dyes are obsolete and nanoparticles are widely used for the labeling and detection for their superior optical property such as highly bright fluorescence, wide excitation and emission wavelength, *etc.* The recent development of nanotechnology has opened up a new horizon of fluorescence detection methods [3]. One of the methods of fluorescence-based detection is FLISA.

FLISA (Fluorescence-Linked Immunosorbent Assay)

ELISA is a method widely used in the area of medical research. It is used for the quantification of antigens in a sample of study. In this method, antibodies are tagged with enzymes that directly or indirectly bind with the antigen. The linked enzyme acts as a catalyst that cleaves the chromogenic substance. The visible color is then detected by a colorimetric detection device [4].

However, in FLISA, a fluorescence-linked antibody is used for detection. The fluorescence that is emitted is measured by a multiplate reader. FLISA can detect more than one target if two or more different antibodies are labeled with different fluorescent colors.

The fluorescence that was used has a limited extinction coefficient and quantum yield but on the other hand, the use of nanoparticles having unique optical properties has a promising prospect in the area of diagnostics. Fluorescence-based sensing of using nanoparticles has revealed a new approach in medical science. Quantum dot and silica nanoparticles are the focus of fluorescence-based sensing (Fig. **1**).

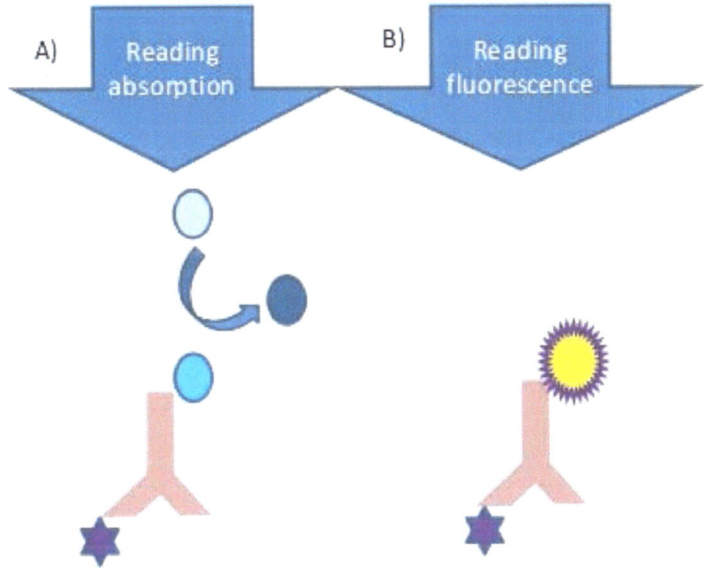

Fig. (1). Schematic diagram of **A)** ELISA, **B)** FLISA.

Quantum dots

Quantum dot fluorophores have significant advantages above the conventional fluorescent markers available in the market. They have controllable size, high sensitivity, stable fluorescence, broad excitation spectra and there is no need for lasers to view the target. Quantum dots have a wide variety of applications in diagnostic medicine and also diagnostic with therapeutics [5]. The main difference between quantum dots and the nanoparticles is that quantum dots are much smaller than the nanoparticles that are 8 to 100 nm in size.

The advantages of quantum dots in the application of diagnostics are as follows:

• Quantum dots are brighter than the other organic fluorophores available.

• The emission peak of the quantum dots are sharp, narrow and with little overlap so they are easier to spot [6].

• The photo bleaching doesn't affect the inorganic quantum dot so they are suitable for *in vivo* applications [7].

• The absorption spectra of quantum dots are wide in contrast to the organic dyes that have very narrow absorption spectra.

However, quantum dots are a promising area for diagnostic applications but there are several, hurdles that need to be addressed before it can be used in full-fledged manner. The hurdles for the application of quantum dots are as follows:

• Many quantum dot nanoparticles contain toxic metals such as cadmium, selenium *etc.* that needs to be coated to meet the requirement of biocompatibility.

• The organic dyes have a size of 0.5nm diameter but quantum dots have a diameter of 6nm-60nm that hinders them to be excreted through the kidney.

• The surface chemistry of the quantum dots largely depends upon the synthesis method that is difficult to control to maintain the consistency.

• There are hurdles in the manufacturing of quantum dots as they vary from batch to batch and do not have the consistency of characteristics of the material.

Fluorescent Silica Nanoparticles

when silica nanoparticles are doped with fluorescence dye they can be used for the detection of pathogens, proteins and nucleic acids. These nanoparticles have the following advantages [8]:

• Silica nanoparticles are abundantly available in the nature.

• They are highly biocompatible in their characteristics.

• High surface to volume ratio helps to bind strongly with the biomolecules.

• High dye-molecule labeling ratio increases the amplification of signals.

• Have control over the wide size range and solubility.

The disadvantages associated with the use of silica nanoparticle in diagnostics are as follows:

• These nanoparticles tend to aggregate more.

• They have a significant amount of nonspecific binding tendency.

Fluorescence Resonance Energy Transfer (FRET)

FRET is a very sensitive and simple method of detection in modern day medicine. FRET donor or accepters are the organic dye conjugated with nanoparticles. It offers a more sensitive flexible platform for bio sensing (Fig. **2**).

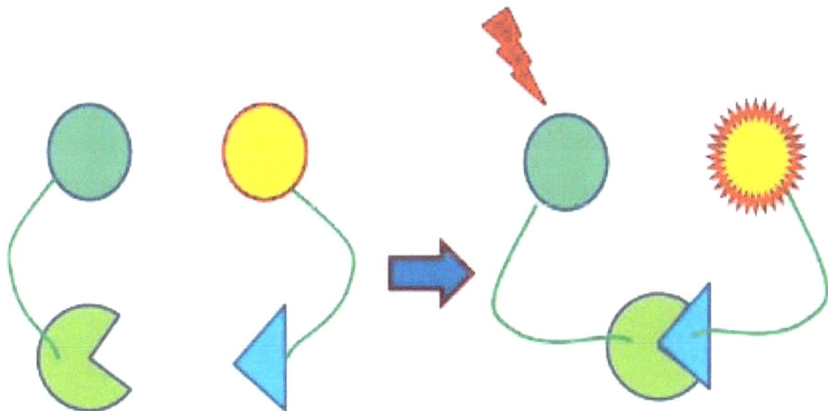

Fig. (2). Schematic diagram of FRET.

Gold nanoparticles, gold nanoparticles are the nonmolecular chromophores that have excellent light collection ability. They are widely used in fluorescent energy transfer (FRET) based assays. The advantages of this type of nanoparticle are as follows:

• Gold nanoparticles have an exceptional quenching ability that makes them a suitable energy accepter for the FRET assays.

• The method is highly fast and easy procedure than other methods [9].

• The procedure is simple and rapid method [10].

The drawbacks of using gold nanoparticle as a chromophore are as follows:

• Gold nanoparticles have significant amount of toxicity within the cell.

• The expense of gold nanoparticle use is high.

Quantum dots, Quantum dote is widely used energy donor in bioassays of FRET. The advantages of this nanoparticle used in FRET are as follows:

• The broad absorption and narrow emission spectra makes this nanoparticle unique in their function.

• The particle size can be controlled and overlapping of the absorption and emission spectra can be adjusted.

• For simplifying the assay design the quantum dot nanoparticles can be conjugated with multiple fluorophores for higher efficiency [11].

Silica nanoparticles, in FRET based biosensing method silica can be used in two different methods. The first one is to use them as solid support and the other way is to dope the fluorescent dyes in the silica nanoparticle. The advantages of the use of silica nanoparticle are as follows:

- The silica nanoparticles are easily separable while preparation.
- The surface modification can be optimized of silica nanoparticles.
- They are hydrophilic.
- They are highly biocompatible [12].

Other Fluorescence Based Detection Methods

Quenching with carbon nanotubes, carbon nanotubes are another type of nanoparticle that is used for fluorescence based detection. The advantages are as follows:

- Single walled carbon nanotubes have superior quenching efficiency for a variety of fluorophores.
- They have low background and high signal to noise ratio [13].

Colorimetric Detection

Colorimetric analysis technique is a method of determination of chemical element or chemical compounds in a solution with the help of color reagent that may be nanoparticles in our example. Nanoparticles that interact with the analytes may change the color of the solution that can be recognized with the naked eye without using expensive instruments. By using this method ion, proteins, peptides and also nucleic acids can be detected [14]. Gold nanoparticles help in the colorimetric detection method.

Gold nanoparticle, spherical gold nanoparticles exhibit different color depending upon their size [15]. The colorimetric detection of metal ions may be achieved by the incorporation of chelating agent on the surface of the gold nanoparticle (Fig. **3**). Gold nanoparticles can also be used for the detection of heavy metal ions as they are highly important in the environmental perspective. These nanoparticles can be used as a sensor of variety of proteins as they change color in the presence of agglutinin, a bivalent lectin etc [16, 17]. Oligonucleotide-functionalized gold nanoparticle also has a potential to detect DNA in a solution [18, 19].

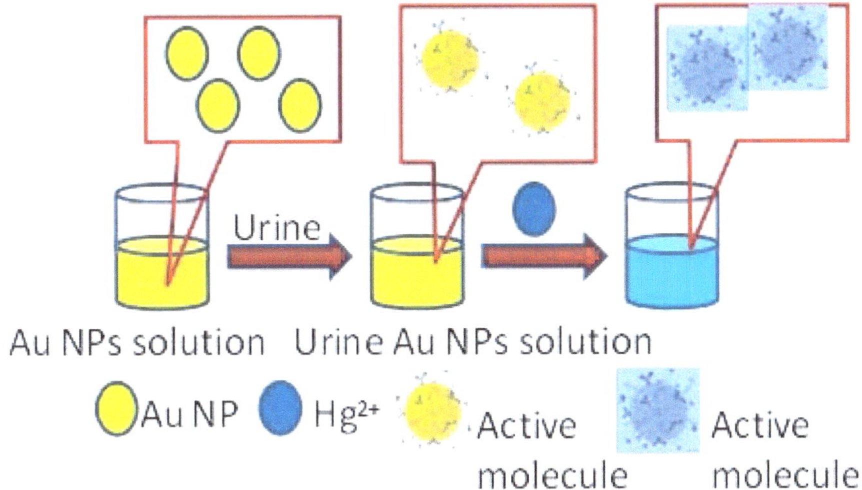

Fig. (3). Schematic of the colorimetric detection of Hg2+ based on simply mixing urine and gold nanoparticles (AuNPs). The active components (uric acid and creatinine) in urine decorated on AuNPs are the reason for selectively binding Hg2+, leading to the aggregation of gold nanoparticles and thereby causing a visual color change.

In addition to the gold nanoparticle some other nanoparticles such as silver nanoparticle, magnetic nanoparticles etc also help in the detection of wide variety of organic and inorganic molecules [20, 21].

Microarray Detection

Microarray is a miniaturized device for the identification of mutated gene, DNA or protein. For detection of DNA in microarray method several alternative nanoparticles have been identified. Gold and silver nanoparticles are used for this purpose [22].

Gold nanoparticles, gold nanoparticles that are larger than 40nm are commonly used as they are readily detected on the visible wavelength. These particles when smaller than 40nm is preferred as they have increased specificity and reactivity. The small gold nanoparticles functionalized with oligonucleotides exhibit high thermal denaturation profile but they barely interact with light. However the optical property can be improved by silver staining enhancement technique. Presently, several companies are developing nanospheres that comprises of DNA probes and gold nanoparticles. These functional nanoparticles are hybridized in cDNA that have 1,000 times more sensitivity than fluorescence [23].

Silver nanoparticle, silver crystals are much larger than gold nanoparticles. Sometimes gold nanoparticles need silver enhancement for growing them to the visible size. Silver deposited around the gold nanoparticles increases its specificity many times than a fluorescent counterpart [24, 25].

Magnetic-Based Detection

Nanoscale magnetic materials are not found in the biological system. So, these nanoparticles can be used as a sensor for targeting specific organ. They have variety of applications as sensors for diagnostic purposes. Magnetic nanoparticles may be detected by several methods in the biological system such as NMR, MRI *etc.*

Magnetic Resonance Imaging (MRI)

Nanoparticle based MRI have received much attention from past decade. Nanoparticle based contrast agents have increased the resolution and sensitivity of the MRI in biomedical applications. Superparamagnetic iron oxide nanoparticles (SPIONs) have increased the sensitivity of the MRI to large extent. Several contrast agents have developed and gained popularity rapidly. The contrast of the contrast agent may be turned “on” or “off” by radiofrequency saturation.

Dendrimers

Dendrimers are synthetic polymer that is fabricated as a core of gadolinium contrast agent.

Liposomes

Liposomes are natural of synthetic lipid nanoparticles that may carry gadolinium either on the surface or as a core component.

Quantum Dots

The inorganic nanoparticle incorporating gadolinium acts as a multifunctional agent for MRI as well as fluorescence microscopy.

Silica Nanoparticle

mesoporous silica have high loading capacity can embed gadolinium in it. This is a promising agent for intravascular MR imaging and soft tissue.

Superparamagnetic Iron Oxide Nanoparticles

Iron oxide nanoparticles are promising contrasting agent for MRI. However they are highly biodegradable that are cleared by macrophages and degraded by lysosome and recycled for the production of red blood cells [26].

Gadolinium Nanoparticle

Gadolinium acts as a contrasting medium to increase the clarity of the image of the internal structure of the body in MRI scan. This helps in the diagnosis of the disease by identifying the blood vessels, inflammation, tumor and small organs in our body. Moreover, this agent is considered to be safe in application of MRI scan [27, 28].

Nuclear Magnetic Resonance (NMR)

Use of magnetic nanoparticle helps in the diagnosis, follow-up and treatment of particular disease condition. These nanoparticles enhance sensitivity and reduce sample preparation steps. The NMR based diagnostic procedure is named as diagnostic magnetic resonance (DMR). DNA, RNA, protein, small molecules such as drugs, bacteria, tumor cells etc are quantified by this method. Magnetic nanoparticles have tremendous potential in the field of biomedical diagnostic applications. For the DMR application the magnetic nanoparticles should have following characteristics [29]:

• The nanoparticles should have superparamagnetic properties.

• Should be highly stable in aqueous media and without the property of aggregation.

• Should have high magnetization and transverse relaxivity.

• With good surfaces chemistry.

Followings are the magnetic nanoparticles that can be used for DMR application:

Cross-linked Iron Oxide Nanoparticles

Cross linked iron oxide nanoparticles are potential application of DMR due to their excellent biocompatibility and stability [30]. These nanoparticles comprises of superparamagnetic iron core composed of maghemite (γ-Fe_2O_3) and/or ferromagnetic magnetite (Fe_3O_4). The core is coated with biocompatible dextran. This structure of the nanoparticle makes them highly biocompatible so that they may be used in a biological system.

Doped-ferrite Nanoparticles

ferrite nanoparticles magnetization can be enhanced by doping them with ferromagnetic elements such as cobalt (Co), manganese (Mn) or nickel (Ni) [31]. At room temperature, the saturation magnetization increases with increasing crystal size up to certain level [32].

Elemental Iron-based Nanoparticles

Iron based nanoparticle and their aqueous solution is a major goal of biomagnetic nano-engineering. Elemental iron have more magnetization than that of metal oxides [33]. The drawback of using elemental iron nanoparticles are that they are highly reactive and subject to rapid oxidation. So, for using them they need to be protected within a shell to maintain their magnetic property. 'Cannonball' was developed for DMR application using Fe-core and ferrite shell magnetic nanoparticle [34].

Electrochemical-Based Detection

The electrical current generated from the oxidative and reductive reactions are identified by electrochemical based detection method. These biosensors have metal and metal oxide detecting electrodes. The detectors have simple and compact electronics with portable instrument. Nanoparticles are extensively studied in the area of electrochemical analysis for its high potential of application in this field [35]. Nanoparticles have exceptional ability against denaturation, stability, ease of mass production, lower cost and ease of bioconjugation they have widespread attention on biosensors that detect DNA and immunosensors [36]. Several nanoparticles are used for electrochemical detection method as follows:

Gold Nanoparticles

Gold nanoparticles have several advantages as they are simple to synthesis, controlled size distribution, optical and electrochemical properties that makes them unique for their utilization in electrochemical detection method. Use of gold nanoparticle in DNA electrochemical assays are widely exploited in the last few years [37]. They are also used extensively in the field of immune assays.

Silver Nanoparticle

The excellent electroactivity of silver nanoparticles make them a highly potential particle for biomedical diagnostics. The findings of silver nanoparticles opened the way for the development of simple and cost-effective electrochemical biosensors [38].

Quantum Dot Nanoparticles

Quantum dot nanoparticles are semiconductor that makes them the most studied nanoparticle in today's world. The normal core/shell structure of this nanoparticle makes them stable structured and stable functionalization [39].

Cerium oxide nanoparticles (CeO_2 NPs)

Cerium oxide nanoparticle is a metal oxide based nanoparticle that has special property as catalyst. In their crystal structure they have many vacancy of oxygen as a result they have high oxygen storage capacity [40]. So, cerium oxide nanoparticle acts as a biosensing agent for their above mentioned properties.

Mercury Selenide Nanoparticles (HgSe NPs)

The electrochemical behavior of mercury selenide nanoparticles were studied from 1960 using mercury electrodes [41]. Simple, sensitive quantification of this nanoparticle opens the area of biosensing by the help of this particle. It has great potential for the further application in electrochemical immunoassays.

Copper-based Nanoparticles (CuNPs)

Copper based metallic nanoparticles have extensively studied for their biocompatible, low toxicity and optical properties. DNA-templated copper nanoparticle is considered as a functional probe for bioanalysis. The microRNAs are also detected by using copper nanoparticles that have ultra-low level detection in the blood sample [42].

Plasmonics-Based Detection

Plasmonic nanoparticles have been developed for sensitive analytical method in the field of biomedical science [43]. Electromagnetic radiation induces the oscillation of surface conduction electrons that is known as surface plasmons. Excitation of surface plasmons leads to the formation of enhanced electromagnetic field at the place of nanoparticle. The techniques used for the detection of this oscillation are surface-enhanced Raman scattering (SERS), surface enhanced infra-red absorption (SEIRA), and metal enhanced fluorescence (MEF).

Surface-Enhanced Raman Scattering (SERS)

The best example of surface plasmon resonance is the optical biosensors. The optical detectable tag can be formed by the surface enhanced Raman Scattering. This system can detect biological species and chemical agents easily. Target genes can also be detected by the help of advanced technology of surface enhanced Raman gene. The nanoprobes formed by this method are highly effective in bio sensing technology [5].

Surface-Enhanced Infrared Absorption (SEIRA)

Hartstein *et al.* first described about the surface enhanced infrared absorption technique [44]. They found that when a bio film is covered by gold and silver nanoparticles there is a significant increase in the absorption level. A high amount of chemical interaction and electric field enhancement results into this above mentioned condition. SEIRA spectroscopy is commonly used for the detection of the electrochemical change.

Metal Enhanced Fluorescence (MEF)

Noble metal nanoparticles enhance fluorescence [45]. Surface plasmon excited in the nanoparticles leads to the formation of this fluorescence. A local electromagnetic field results in to the oscillation and emission of this fluorescence. This phenomenon is known as metal-enhanced fluorescence (MEF) (Table **1** and **2**) [46].

Table 1. Brief discussion about different materials.

Name and size	Description	Applications	Advantages	Disadvantages
Quantum dots (2-10nm)	Semiconductor nanocrystal with unique spectral property Core shell quantum dot with high biocompatibility and conjugation ability	*In vitro* detection of protein, toxin and DNA *In vivo* detection of mRNAs	Highly bright than organic fluorophores Greater photostability and extinction coefficient Broad excitation spectra and tunable emission spectra.	Difficult to prepare. Undefined toxicity
Doped silica nanoparticle (20-70nm)	Multiple fluorophores doped in silica matrix Diagnosis using FRET	*In vitro* detection of bacteria and antibodies Optical and magnetic imaging	Biocompatible and hydrophilic in nature Highly brighter than fluorophores Easy preparation and surface modification	Nanoparticle size and intensity compromise each other Accurate and reproducible dye loading ratio is needed
Microbeads with optically encoded (1-10μm)	Identifiable features with coding element	*In vitro* detection Drug discovery Diagnosis of diseases	Large information may be procured	Quality control is needed Separate fluorophore is needed Large size not suitable of many applications

(Table 1) cont.....

Name and size	Description	Applications	Advantages	Disadvantages
SERS probe (30-100nm)	Metallic nanoparticle for Raman spectroscopy	*In vitro* detection of DNA and protein	Narrow Raman spectroscopic lines and broad spectral window	Specialized equipment is needed Hard to use on commercial scale
Metallic barcode (diameter: 0.3μm)	Cylindrical shaped metallic nanoparticle	Used for sandwich immunoassays and SNP analysis	Large barcoding library May be used with conventional light microscope	Particles may break Aggregation may occur Complicated manufacturing procedure

Table 2. Main features of the most relevant imaging modalities.

Technique	Source of radiation	Advantages	Disadvantages
MRI	Radio waves	High spatial resolution; good contrast; functional information	Low sensitivity; expensive equipment
CT	X-rays	Good anatomical information	Poor contrast, uses ionizing radiation; expensive equipment
PET	High-energy γ rays	High sensitivity; provides biochemical information	Low resolution; requires radio nucleotides; expensive equipment
SPECT	Lower energy γ rays	High sensitivity	Low resolution; requires radio nucleotides; expensive equipment
Optical imaging	Visible light	Inexpensive equipment; allow monitorization of several events	Limited anatomical resolution; low sensitivity of deep imaging
Ultrasound	High frequency sound	Inexpensive equipment	Low resolution

CONCLUSION

Nanoscience and nanotechnology are fields of the same team. The fabrication of a proper nanoparticle that can be used for the medical field needs not only the scientists of nanotechnology but also material scientists, biotechnologists, clinicians and end-users. Nanoparticles should have several characteristics for using them as a diagnostic of different disease conditions. They should be biocompatible without any toxic effect on health; their particle size should be optimum; when used through intravenous injection, they should not have any antigen-antibody reaction, *etc.* In this chapter, we intended to find out different diagnostic tools that are explored in the recent past using nanoparticles for the diagnosis of divers' disease conditions.

In closing, we can say that the potential uses of nanoparticles are yet to be revealed in the health care sector. Optimum standardization and characterization of the nanoparticles are true hurdles in this technology.

REFERENCES

[1] Laurentius LB, Owens NA, Park J, Crawford AC, Porter MD. Advantages and limitations of nanoparticle labeling for early diagnosis of infection. Expert Rev Mol Diagn 2016; 16(8): 883-95. [http://dx.doi.org/10.1080/14737159.2016.1205489] [PMID: 27337490]

[2] Wang L, O'Donoghue MB, Tan W. Nanoparticles for multiplex diagnostics and imaging. Nanomedicine (Lond) 2006; 1(4): 413-26. [http://dx.doi.org/10.2217/17435889.1.4.413] [PMID: 17716144]

[3] Zhong W. Nanomaterials in fluorescence-based biosensing. Anal Bioanal Chem 2009; 394(1): 47-59. [http://dx.doi.org/10.1007/s00216-009-2643-x]

[4] Gan SD, Patel KR. Enzyme immunoassay and enzyme-linked immunosorbent assay. J Invest Dermatol 2013; 133(9): e12. [http://dx.doi.org/10.1038/jid.2013.287] [PMID: 23949770]

[5] Jain KK. Applications of nanobiotechnology in clinical diagnostics. Clin Chem 2007; 53(11): 2002-9. [http://dx.doi.org/10.1373/clinchem.2007.090795] [PMID: 17890442]

[6] Resch-Genger U, Grabolle M, Cavaliere-Jaricot S, Nitschke R, Nann T. Quantum dots *versus* organic dyes as fluorescent labels. Nat Methods 2008; 5(9): 763-75. [http://dx.doi.org/10.1038/nmeth.1248] [PMID: 18756197]

[7] Beloglazova NV, Speranskaya ES, Wu A, *et al.* Novel multiplex fluorescent immunoassays based on quantum dot nanolabels for mycotoxins determination. Biosens Bioelectron 2014; 62: 59-65. [http://dx.doi.org/10.1016/j.bios.2014.06.021] [PMID: 24976152]

[8] Tang L, Cheng J. Nonporous silica nanoparticles for nanomedicine application. Nano Today 2013; 8(3): 290-312. [http://dx.doi.org/10.1016/j.nantod.2013.04.007] [PMID: 23997809]

[9] Ray PC, Fortner A, Darbha GK. Gold Nanoparticle Based FRET Asssay for the Detection of DNA Cleavage. J Phys Chem B 2006 110(42): 20745-8. [http://dx.doi.org/10.1021/jp065121l]

[10] Shi J, Tian F, Lyu J, Yang M. Nanoparticle based fluorescence resonance energy transfer (FRET) for biosensing applications. J Mater Chem B Mater Biol Med 2015; 3(35): 6989-7005. [http://dx.doi.org/10.1039/C5TB00885A] [PMID: 32262700]

[11] Curutchet C, Franceschetti A, Zunger A, Scholes GD. Examining förster energy transfer for semiconductor nanocrystalline quantum dot donors and acceptors. J Phys Chem C. 2008; 112(35): 13336-41. [http://dx.doi.org/10.1021/jp805682m]

[12] Wang L, Tan W. Multicolor FRET silica nanoparticles by single wavelength excitation. Nano Lett 2006; 6(1): 84-8.

[http://dx.doi.org/10.1021/nl052105b] [PMID: 16402792]

[13] Zhu Z, Yang R, You M, Zhang X, Wu Y, Tan W. Single-walled carbon nanotube as an effective quencher. Anal Bioanal Chem 2009; 396: 73-83.

[14] Jazayeri MH, Aghaie T, Avan A, Vatankhah A, Ghaffari MRS. Colorimetric detection based on gold nano particles (GNPs): An easy, fast, inexpensive, low-cost and short time method in detection of analytes (protein, DNA, and ion). Sensing and Bio-Sensing Research. 2018; 20: 1-8.

[15] Jain PK, Lee KS, El-Sayed IH, El-Sayed MA. Calculated absorption and scattering properties of gold nanoparticles of different size, shape, and composition: applications in biological imaging and biomedicine. J. Phys. Chem. B. 2006; 110(14): 7238-48.

[16] Otsuka H, Akiyama Y, Nagasaki Y, Kataoka K. Quantitative and reversible lectin-induced association of gold nanoparticles modified with α-Lactosyl-ω-mercapto-poly(ethylene glycol). J Am Chem Soc 2001; 123(34): 8226-30.

[17] Tsai C-S, Yu T-B, Chen C-T. Gold nanoparticle-based competitive colorimetric assay for detection of protein-protein interactions. Chem Commun (Camb) 2005; (34): 4273-5. [http://dx.doi.org/10.1039/b507237a] [PMID: 16113719]

[18] Mirkin CA, Letsinger RL, Mucic RC, Storhoff JJ. A DNA-based method for rationally assembling nanoparticles into macroscopic materials. Nature 1996; 382(6592): 607-9. [http://dx.doi.org/10.1038/382607a0] [PMID: 8757129]

[19] Elghanian R, Storhoff JJ, Mucic RC, Letsinger RL, Mirkin CA. Selective colorimetric detection of polynucleotides based on the distance-dependent optical properties of gold nanoparticles. Science 1997; 277(5329): 1078-81. [http://dx.doi.org/10.1126/science.277.5329.1078] [PMID: 9262471]

[20] Zhou Y, Zhao H, He Y, Ding N, Cao Q. Colorimetric detection of Cu_{2+} using 4-mercaptobenzoic acid modified silver nanoparticles. Colloids Surf, A Physicochem Eng Asp 2011; 391(1): 179-83.

[21] Su L, Feng J, Zhou X, Ren C, Li H, Chen X. Colorimetric detection of urine glucose based $ZnFe_2O_4$ magnetic nanoparticles. Anal Chem 2012; 84(13): 5753-8. [http://dx.doi.org/10.1021/ac300939z]

[22] Festag G, Steinbrück A, Wolff A, Csaki A, Möller R, Fritzsche W. Optimization of gold nanoparticle-based DNA detection for microarrays. J Fluoresc 2005; 15(2): 161-70. [http://dx.doi.org/10.1007/s10895-005-2524-4] [PMID: 15883771]

[23] Zhang YQ, Wang YF, Jiang XD. The application of nanoparticles in biochips. Recent Pat Biotechnol 2008; 2(1): 55-9. [http://dx.doi.org/10.2174/187220808783330938] [PMID: 19075853]

[24] Storhoff JJ, Marla SS, Bao P, *et al.* Gold nanoparticle-based detection of genomic DNA targets on microarrays using a novel optical detection system. Biosens Bioelectron 2004; 19(8): 875-83. [http://dx.doi.org/10.1016/j.bios.2003.08.014] [PMID: 15128107]

[25] Pedroso S, Guillen IA. Microarray and nanotechnology applications of functional nanoparticles. Comb Chem High Throughput Screen 2006; 9(5): 389-97. [http://dx.doi.org/10.2174/138620706777452438] [PMID: 16787152]

[26] Mao X, Xu J, Cui H. Functional nanoparticles for magnetic resonance imaging. Wiley Interdiscip Rev Nanomed Nanobiotechnol 2016; 8(6): 814-41. [http://dx.doi.org/10.1002/wnan.1400] [PMID: 27040463]

[27] Do C, DeAguero J, Brearley A, Trejo X, Howard T, Escobar GP, *et al.* Gadolinium-based contrast agent use, their safety, and practice evolution. Kidney 360 2020; 1(6): 561-8.

[28] Mitsumori LM, Bhargava P, Essig M, Maki JH. Magnetic resonance imaging using gadolinium-based contrast agents. Top Magn Reson Imaging 2014; 23(1): 51-69.

[http://dx.doi.org/10.1097/RMR.0b013e31829c4686] [PMID: 24477166]

[29] Shao H, Yoon TJ, Liong M, Weissleder R, Lee H. Magnetic nanoparticles for biomedical NMR-based diagnostics. Beilstein J Nanotechnol 2010; 1: 142-54. [http://dx.doi.org/10.3762/bjnano.1.17] [PMID: 21977404]

[30] Perez JM, Josephson L, O'Loughlin T, Högemann D, Weissleder R. Magnetic relaxation switches capable of sensing molecular interactions. Nat Biotechnol 2002; 20(8): 816-20. [http://dx.doi.org/10.1038/nbt720] [PMID: 12134166]

[31] Jun YW, Lee JH, Cheon J. Chemical design of nanoparticle probes for high-performance magnetic resonance imaging. Angew Chem Int Ed Engl 2008; 47(28): 5122-35. [http://dx.doi.org/10.1002/anie.200701674] [PMID: 18574805]

[32] Smolensky ED, Park H-YE, Zhou Y, *et al.* Scaling laws at the nano size: the effect of particle size and shape on the magnetism and relaxivity of iron oxide nanoparticle contrast agents. J Mater Chem B Mater Biol Med 2013; 1(22): 2818-28. [http://dx.doi.org/10.1039/c3tb00369h] [PMID: 23819021]

[33] Miguel OB, Gossuin Y, Morales MP, Gillis P, Muller RN, Veintemillas-Verdaguer S. Comparative analysis of the 1H NMR relaxation enhancement produced by iron oxide and core-shell iron-iron oxide nanoparticles. Magn Reson Imag 2007; 25(10): 1437-41.

[34] Lee H, Yoon TJ, Weissleder R. Ultrasensitive detection of bacteria using core-shell nanoparticles and an NMR-filter system. Angew Chem Int Ed Engl 2009; 48(31): 5657-60. [http://dx.doi.org/10.1002/anie.200901791] [PMID: 19554581]

[35] Liu CC. Electrochemical based biosensors. Biosensors (Basel) 2012; 2(3): 269-72. [http://dx.doi.org/10.3390/bios2030269] [PMID: 25585929]

[36] Iglesias-Mayor A, Amor-Gutiérrez O, Costa-García A, de la Escosura-Muñiz A. Nanoparticles as emerging labels in electrochemical immunosensors. Sensors (Basel) 2019; 19(23): 5137. [http://dx.doi.org/10.3390/s19235137] [PMID: 31771201]

[37] Maduraiveeran G, Sasidharan M, Ganesan V. Electrochemical sensor and biosensor platforms based on advanced nanomaterials for biological and biomedical applications. Biosens. Bioelectron 2018; 103: 113-29. [http://dx.doi.org/10.1016/j.bios.2017.12.031]

[38] Tschulik K, Batchelor-McAuley C, Toh H-S, Stuart EJE, Compton RG. Electrochemical studies of silver nanoparticles: a guide for experimentalists and a perspective. Phys Chem Chem Phys 2014; 16(2): 616-23. [http://dx.doi.org/10.1039/C3CP54221A] [PMID: 24247993]

[39] Grabolle M, Ziegler J, Merkulov A, Nann T, Resch-Genger U. Stability and fluorescence quantum yield of CdSe-ZnS quantum dots-influence of the thickness of the ZnS shell. Ann N Y Acad Sci 2008; 1130: 235-41. [http://dx.doi.org/10.1196/annals.1430.021] [PMID: 18596353]

[40] Campbell CT, Peden CHF. Chemistry oxygen vacancies and catalysis on ceria surfaces. Science 2005; 309(5735): 713-4. [http://dx.doi.org/10.1126/science.1113955] [PMID: 16051777]

[41] Mathe MK, Cox SM, Venkatasamy V, Happek U, Stickney JL. Formation of HgSe thin films using electrochemical atomic layer epitaxy. J Electrochem Soc 2005; 152(11): C751. [http://dx.doi.org/10.1149/1.2047547]

[42] Wang Y, Zhang X, Zhao L, Bao T, Wen W, Zhang X, *et al.* Integrated amplified aptasensor with in-situ precise preparation of copper nanoclusters for ultrasensitive electrochemical detection of microRNA 21. Biosens. Bioelectron 2017; 98: 386-91.

[43] Martines-Arano H, García-Pérez BE, Vidales-Hurtado MA, Trejo-Valdez M, Hernández-Gómez LH, Torres-Torres C. Chaotic signatures exhibited by plasmonic effects in AU nanoparticles with cells.

Sensors (Basel) 2019; 19(21): 4728.
[http://dx.doi.org/10.3390/s19214728] [PMID: 31683534]

[44] Hartstein A, Kirtley JR, Tsang JC. Enhancement of the infrared absorption from molecular monolayers with thin metal overlayers. Phys Rev Lett 1980; 45(3): 201-4.
[http://dx.doi.org/10.1103/PhysRevLett.45.201]

[45] Lim WQ, Gao Z. Plasmonic nanoparticles in biomedicine. Nano Today 2016; 11(2): 168-88.
[http://dx.doi.org/10.1016/j.nantod.2016.02.002]

[46] Krajczewski J, Kołątaj K, Kudelski A. Plasmonic nanoparticles in chemical analysis. RSC Advances 2017; 7(28): 17559-76.
[http://dx.doi.org/10.1039/C7RA01034F]

CHAPTER 4

Drug Delivery through Nanoparticle in Treatment of Diseases

Abstract: The study of nanocarriers for drug delivery opens a novel platform for the development of delivery vehicles that can transport and control release the payload in the target disease tissue by the smart application of biotechnology and nanotechnology. This study highlights the parameters that can be fabricated to make the nanocarrier optimum for specific disease condition and their current clinical application areas. Moreover, this study also reports about the several organic and inorganic nanoparticles and their properties that make them unique as a drug delivery vehicle. Despite remarkable development in this area of application, nanocarriers demonstrate a significant amount of unwanted side effects, such as, cytotoxicity or off-target side effects that diminish their efficiency in the biotechnology and biomedical applications. A complex biological environment makes this field more complicated, so, deep knowledge of the biological condition is the most important before developing an optimum therapeutic solution.

Keywords: Alginate, Cancer, Carbon nanotube, Cellulose, Chitosan, Dendrimer, Drug delivery vehicle, Gold nanoparticle, HIV, Inorganic nanoparticle, Liposome, Nanomedicine, Nutraceuticals, Organic nanoparticle, Polymeric nanoparticle, Quantum dot, Silica nanoparticle, Surface chemistry, Xanthan gum.

INTRODUCTION

Currently, wide research and development are taking place in the area of biotechnology and Nanomedicines. Nanomedicines are making significant advancement in the area of disease diagnosis and drug delivery. Optimum engineered nanoparticles are the main tool for this advancement. Nanoparticles have a wide possibility in the field of drug delivery as they have some unique properties such as high surface to volume ratio, their ability to carry large molecules *i.e.,* DNA, RNA, proteins, drugs, *etc.* These nanoparticles may be engineered so that they can have reduced cytotoxicity and increased carrying capacity for drugs. The source material of these nanoparticles may be of biological origin such as lipid, lactic acid , chitosan or chemical in origin such as silica, gold or

Rituparna Acharya

polymers. These nanostructures help to deliver drugs to the target organ and help to reduce the dosage and side effects that are experienced by traditional medicines.

In this study, we intend to discuss the nanoparticles that are used as a nanocarrier for the delivery of drugs and will focus on the main characteristics that may be fabricated to make them unique for a specific application. We will analyze the main parameters that influence the physicochemical property of the delivery vehicle. Further, we will discuss the current field of application of these nanocarriers in several disease conditions and various types of nanocarriers and their properties in this field.

CHARACTERISTICS OF NANOPARTICLE FOR THE FABRICATION OF DRUG DELIVERY VEHICLE

Before going into the fact of what will be an ideal nanoparticle for the delivery of drugs into the human system, we must know what are the hurdles faced by the scientists for producing a nanoparticle that is optimum for our system. There are mainly three different routes of administration of nanoparticles in a human body *i.e.*, through injection, inhalation and through oral route. Before the distribution of nanoparticles in different organs, the main consideration is the interaction of particle proteins in the systemic circulation [1, 2]. If in the systemic circulation the nanoparticles are recognized as an antigen, then antigen-antibody reaction takes place and if they are recognized as foreign particles, they are engulfed by macrophages in the circulatory system. However, these above-mentioned reactions may be influenced by the size and surface characteristics of the nanoparticles [3] that will be elaborated in the following sections:

Size of Nanoparticles

The size and shape of the nanoparticles affect their efficiency and target ability on the target organ. These parameters affect how the macrophage and other cells "see" them in the body and whether the antigen-antibody reactions will develop or not when they are exposed to the systemic circulation. Due to their minute particle size, the nanoparticles can cross the blood-brain barrier (BBB) [4].

The drug release efficiency is the next important matter in the optimum development of the nanoparticles [5]. Due to the smaller size, the surface area to volume ratio increases that leads to the situation of drug molecules closer to the nanoparticle, which in turn leads to faster release of the drug [6].

Moreover, the optimum size of nanoparticles is less than 100nm. If the size somehow increases to 200nm, it activates the lymphatic system and clearance of nanoparticles from the circulation becomes quicker [7].

Surface Property of Nanoparticles

The surface properties of nanoparticles are an important parameter for the development of an ideal nanoparticle [8]. The hydrophobic property of the surface of nanoparticles makes them more inclined to the clearance of nanoparticles from the blood circulation [9]. Making the surface of the nanoparticle hydrophilic enhances their time in circulation.

Moreover, one more problem still remains for the small nanoparticles that have large surface area *i.e.*, the problem of aggregation. Several strategies are employed to overcome this problem such as using a capping agent to change their zeta potential [10].

From the above theories it can be concluded that the particle size of the nanoparticles should not be small enough to leak from the blood vessels and should not be large enough to be susceptible to macrophage clearance [11].

Drug Loading and Release From the Nanoparticle

Another aspect of ideal nanoparticle development is their optimization depending upon the release of the drug from the matrix. The release of drugs from the nanoparticle depends upon several factors such as, pH, drug solubility, temperature, *etc.* [12]. However, nanocapsules and nanospheres are the two types of formulations that can affect the release of the drugs from the nanoparticle [13, 14].

APPLICATION OF NANOPARTICLES IN DRUG DELIVERY

Cancer Therapy

In today's world, chemotherapy is one of the treatment procedures for cancer. However, this treatment method has several side effects [15]. Chemotherapy is mainly aimed at all the rapidly dividing cells in the body that include hair follicles and intestinal epithelium. In this regard, nanoparticles have a new avenue for targeted therapy. It can target specific cells and avoid the toxic effect of other normal tissues and organs [16].

The nanoparticles such as liposomes, dendrimers and carbon nanotubes are being successfully utilized for the treatment of cancer. Most of these studies are at the clinical trial stage [17]. Several nanoparticles containing different anticancer drugs are targeted for delivery into the tumor cells are under clinical trial [18]

HIV and AIDS Treatment

Acquired immune deficiency syndrome develops due to the infection of the human immunodeficiency virus (HIV) [19]. When the treatment of this disease was first developed, the patient was required to take 30-40 pills a day. However, the research had developed nanoparticles that reduced the count of pills per day to just a few [20].

Antiretroviral therapy is nowadays the most used method for combating HIV infection. A combination of three or more multi drugs is used for the treatment of AIDS that is known as highly effective antiretroviral therapy (HAART) [21].

Nanoparticles have high utility in the delivery of retroviral drugs [22]. They can cross the mucosal epithelium and blood-brain barrier that are necessary for the treatment of AIDS [23].

Nutraceutical Delivery Through Nanoparticles

Nutraceuticals are standardized components that have health benefits and they are actually derived from food. They are used as a complementary of several allopathic medicines and provide health benefits against several disease conditions [24]. Nanoparticles however, provide improved dissolution mechanism to these molecules *via* formulations developed with them [25].

Nutraceuticals have many benefits on our body such as they act as an anti-inflammatory, antiapoptotic, antioxidative and antiangiogenic. Curcumin (diferuloyl methane) is one of the most highly studied nutraceutical that have many benefits. Use of curcumin has several drawbacks such as they are highly water soluble and poorly bioavailable. This issue is addressed by nanoparticles that made them overcome these above said drawbacks [26].

Resveratrol is another most important nutraceutical that have several beneficial activities such as it acts as an antioxidant, anti-inflammatory, cardio protective and anticancer [27]. Nanoformulations of this molecule also increased the pharmacokinetic and bioavailability of this nutraceutical [28].

NANOCARRIERS FOR DRUG DELIVERY

Conventional drugs have critical issues associated with that such as toxicity, poor specificity and induction of drug resistance. Nanocarrier based platforms for the delivery of drugs increases the surface area to volume ratio that leads to the effective and efficient delivery of the drug to the target tissue. The overall goal of the nanocarrier based delivery system is to minimize side effects of the drug.

Modern day nanocarriers can be subdivided into mainly two catagories *i.e.*, inorganic and organic nano structures. The physiochemical properties of these nanparticles can be tuned into by altering their composition, shape, size and surface properties. Many nanocarriers are already approved for treatment and others are in the clinical trial phase [29, 30]. In the following section we are intended to discuss about many nanocarriers and their characteristics.

Organic Polymer Based Nanocarriers

Organic nanocarriers are mainly carbon based nanoparticles that have high biocompatibility and improved drug loading capacity. Their larger size helps in carrying wide variety of drugs incorporated within them [31, 32]. The properties and characteristics of these nanoparticles are discussed as follows:

Chitosan

Chitosan have a wide range of application in nanotechnology because of its highly biocompatible and biodegradable property. Chitosan nanoparticles are tested in parental and non-parenteral routes of administration conjugated with wide variety of drugs [33]. Modified chitosan nanoparticle conjugated with paclitaxel demonstrated improved intestinal pharmacokinetic profile [34]. Experimental results indicated that the use of this nanocarrier improves the bioavailability and increased tumor targeting [35]. Chitosan based nasal formulation morphine is in clinical trial.

Alginate

Alginate is a biopolymer with a wide range of applications. Prolonged and better controlled drug administration has increased the demand for polymeric nanoparticles. Alginate plays a significant role in the controlled release of drugs. Depending upon the pH alginate forms two types of gels *i.e.,* acid gel and ionotropic gel. So far there are 200 different alginate grads and many numbers of salts are prepared. All the various types of alginates are not evaluated fully in their application as pharmaceutical agent but they have a high potential as a delivery vehicle of drugs [36].

Xanthan Gum

Xanthomonas campestris produces xanthan gum that is high molecular weight hetero polysaccharide product. They are highly bio adhesive and because if it's nontoxic, biocompatibility it is widely used in pharmaceuticals [37]. Controlled drug release to the targeted organ can be performed by the use of this biopolymer. Xanthan can entrap drug within the gel and slowly release it to the target organ. Gold nanoparticles synthesized using xanthan makes them nontoxic and highly biocompatible [38].

Cellulose

Cellulose and its derivatives are extensively used in drug delivery to increase its solubility and controlled release of the drug to the organ. Its highly environment friendly and renewable polymer. Various nanocarriers such as bacterial cellulose (BC), microcrystalline cellulose, cellulose acetate, cellulose nanocrystals, carboxymethyl cellulose, cellulose nanofibrills, *etc.* are intensely used in biomedical applications, such as scaffold, tissue engineering, artificial blood vessel, artificial skin, skin grafts, drug carrier, and chronic skin diseases *etc.* however special attention is paid on drug delivery for cancer therapy [39].

Liposomes

Although polymeric nanoparticles have several advantages in biomedical applications, lipid based nanoparticles are still supreme in the market. In the area of biomedical and biotechnology the vesicles composed of natural and synthetic lipid have a wide range of application as a drug delivery vehicle [40, 41]. This lipid based nanocarriers are easy to synthesis than other polymeric nanoparticles. These liposomes are considered to be a better nanocarrier of drugs as their membrane structure is similar to the cell membrane of living cell. As a result they are highly biocompatible and biodegradable and can carry both hydrophobic and hydrophilic drugs as well.

Dendrimers

Dendrimers are polymeric branched compounds that is specifically suited for the drug delivery purpose [42]. The dendritic nature of this nanoparticle allows drugs to bind at the outside surface of the molecule. The specific targeting of this nanoparticle to the target organ is further enhanced by functionalization of the surface by antibodies. Few research publications highlight its toxicity as a delivery vehicle (Fig. **1**) [43].

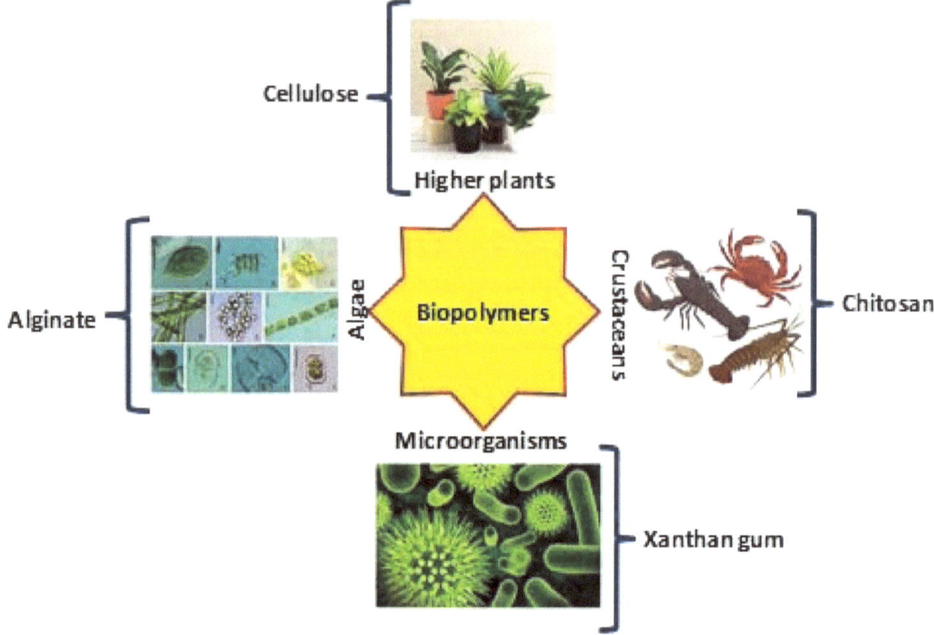

Fig. (1). Sources of natural biopolymers used for the synthesis of nanoparticles.

Inorganic Nanoparticles

Currently there are many inorganic nanoparticles that are employed for drug delivery to the target organ. However, there are some toxicity issues that are addressed in recent research publications. Several metallic nanoparticles have specific properties that help in drug delivery. Bimetallic nanoparticles demonstrate antimicrobial efficiencies in contrast with their monometallic counterparts [44]. In this study we will discuss several inorganic nanocarriers for drug delivery as follows:

Carbon Nanotubes

Carbon nanotubes are biopersistent fibers that may be single walled of multi walled structure. These nanoparticles have unique physiochemical properties and biological characteristics that make them potential drug delivery vehicle. Their nano-needle shape allows them to penetrate through the cell membrane by endocytosis method. Reactivity of carbon nanotube with the biological system is regulated by its size, shape, purity, surface charge chemistry *etc.* Carbon nanotube is mostly studied delivery vehicle for cancer because of its unique physiochemical characteristics and high drug payload, structural flexibility, intrinsic stability, appropriate surface functionalization *etc*. [45, 46].

Gold Nanoparticles

Gold nanoparticles may be synthesized in a wide variety of forms such as rods and dots. They are commercially available in a wide range of sizes and are detectable in low concentrations. They do not have any cytotoxicity and are nontoxic in nature. They may carry a wide variety of genes and drugs for the treatment of cancer and other types of disease conditions [47, 48].

Quantum Dots

Quantum dots are heterogeneous semiconductors and fluorescent nanoparticles that are widely used in biomedical applications [49]. This nanoparticle can act as a delivery vehicle that can control the release or sustain the release of the drug. The released behavior can be achieved by external factors such as light, heat, magnetic fields or radio frequency [50 - 52]. Naked quantum dot nanoparticles are highly toxic by inducing reactive oxygen species and damaging the nucleus, mitochondria and plasma membrane.

Superparamagnetic Iron-Oxide Nanoparticles

Superparamagnetic nanoparticles are proposed successfully as a drug delivery vehicle [53 - 55]. When these magnetic particles are reduced in size upto 10-20nm, they demonstrate super para-magnetic effect. The surface properties of superparamagnetic iron oxide nanoparticles are changed to make them suitable for tagging them with antibodies and binding them with a wide variety of drugs that targets several different organs and targeted therapy for cancer [56]. Although they are highly suitable for drug delivery but because of their effect as altered gene expression profiles, oxidative stress, disturbance in iron homeostasis, and altered cellular responses make them limited in the use in clinical practice.

Silica Nanoparticles

Spherical silica nanoparticles are found to be cytotoxic depending upon their dose and exposure time [57]. On the other hand, mesoporous silica nanoparticles are highly used in biomedical applications because of their simple synthesis method and characteristic porous architecture. They allow loading a large number of drugs and accumulate in the target organ. Mesoporous silica nanoparticles are considered as an attractive nanocarrier for their specific characteristics such as high biocompatibility, high loading capacity for hydrophilic and hydrophobic drugs, large specific surface area, controllable pore diameters and good thermal and chemical stability that make them an ideal drug delivery vehicle. They are used as an effective delivery vehicle for delivering several anticancer drugs such as paclitaxel, doxorubicin, and methotrexate. The controlled release of drugs is triggered by temperature, pH, light, magnetic field, electric and mechanical stimuli, as well as enzyme and chemical reactions [58, 59].

CONCLUSION

In this study, we have highlighted the nanoparticles and their properties that make them unique in biomedical applications as a drug delivery vehicle. The traditional drugs have several drawbacks such as high doses to accomplish specific therapeutic effect and many side effects. However, these nanocarriers when delivering these drugs are highly specific to the target thus reducing dosage and off-target side effects. There are mainly two types of nanocarriers *i.e.,* organic and inorganic nanoparticles that are exploited profitably. Organic nanocarriers are highly biocompatible with less cytotoxicity and better physiochemical properties. On the other hand, inorganic nanocarriers have properties that highly depend upon their size, shape, surface chemistry *etc.*

Although there are a wide variety of nanocarriers invented by scientists, their properties highly fluctuate with the intrinsic properties of the biological environment. These alterations of properties largely influence and complicate the use of nanoparticles in drug delivery. Thus a deep knowledge of the diseased tissue is highly recommended before the development of a therapeutic protocol using nanocarriers [60].

REFERENCES

[1] Mu Q, Jiang G, Chen L, Zhou H, Fourches D, Tropsha A, *et al.* Chemical basis of interactions between engineered nanoparticles and biological systems. Chem Rev 2014; 114(15): 7740-81. [http://dx.doi.org/10.1021/cr400295a]

[2] Prado-Gotor R, Grueso E. A kinetic study of the interaction of DNA with gold nanoparticles: mechanistic aspects of the interaction. Phys Chem Chem Phys 2011; 13(4): 1479-89. [http://dx.doi.org/10.1039/C0CP00901F] [PMID: 21132199]

[3] Alexis F, Pridgen E, Molnar LK, Farokhzad OC. Factors affecting the clearance and biodistribution of polymeric nanoparticles. Mol Pharm 2008; 5(4): 505-15. [http://dx.doi.org/10.1021/mp800051m] [PMID: 18672949]

[4] McMillan J, Batrakova E, Gendelman HE. Cell delivery of therapeutic nanoparticles. Prog Mol Biol Transl Sci 2011; 104: 563-601. [http://dx.doi.org/10.1016/B978-0-12-416020-0.00014-0] [PMID: 22093229]

[5] Chavanpatil MD, Khdair A, Patil Y, Handa H, Mao G, Panyam J. Polymer-surfactant nanoparticles for sustained release of water-soluble drugs. J Pharm Sci 2007; 96(12): 3379-89. [http://dx.doi.org/10.1002/jps.20961] [PMID: 17721942]

[6] Buzea C, Pacheco II, Robbie K. Nanomaterials and nanoparticles: sources and toxicity. Biointerphases 2007; 2(4): MR17-71. [http://dx.doi.org/10.1116/1.2815690] [PMID: 20419892]

[7] Prokop A, Davidson JM. Nanovehicular intracellular delivery systems. J Pharm Sci 2008; 97(9): 3518-90. [http://dx.doi.org/10.1002/jps.21270] [PMID: 18200527]

[8] Bantz C, Koshkina O, Lang T, *et al.* The surface properties of nanoparticles determine the agglomeration state and the size of the particles under physiological conditions. Beilstein J Nanotechnol 2014; 5: 1774-86.
[http://dx.doi.org/10.3762/bjnano.5.188] [PMID: 25383289]

[9] Kou L, Sun J, Zhai Y, He Z. The endocytosis and intracellular fate of nanomedicines: Implication for rational design. Asian J. Pharm. Sci 2013; 8(1): 1-10.

[10] Li D, Kaner RB. Shape and aggregation control of nanoparticles: not shaken, not stirred. J Am Chem Soc 2006; 128(3): 968-75.
[http://dx.doi.org/10.1021/ja056609n] [PMID: 16417388]

[11] Sykes EA, Dai Q, Sarsons CD, *et al.* Tailoring nanoparticle designs to target cancer based on tumor pathophysiology. Proc Natl Acad Sci USA 2016; 113(9): E1142-51.
[http://dx.doi.org/10.1073/pnas.1521265113] [PMID: 26884153]

[12] Son G-H, Lee B-J, Cho C-W. Mechanisms of drug release from advanced drug formulations such as polymeric-based drug-delivery systems and lipid nanoparticles. Int. J. Pharm. Investig 2017; 47(4): 287-96.
[http://dx.doi.org/10.1007/s40005-017-0320-1]

[13] Mora-Huertas CE, Fessi H, Elaissari A. Polymer-based nanocapsules for drug delivery. Int J Pharm 2010; 385(1-2): 113-42.
[http://dx.doi.org/10.1016/j.ijpharm.2009.10.018] [PMID: 19825408]

[14] Lee JH, Yeo Y. Controlled drug release from pharmaceutical nanocarriers. Chem Eng Sci 2015; 125: 75-84.
[http://dx.doi.org/10.1016/j.ces.2014.08.046] [PMID: 25684779]

[15] Baudino TA. Targeted cancer therapy: the next generation of cancer treatment. Curr Drug Discov Technol 2015; 12(1): 3-20.
[http://dx.doi.org/10.2174/1570163812666150602144310] [PMID: 26033233]

[16] Shen B, Ma Y, Yu S, Ji C. Smart multifunctional magnetic nanoparticle-based drug delivery system for cancer thermo-chemotherapy and intracellular imaging. ACS Appl. Mater. Interfaces 2016; 8(37): 24502-8.
[http://dx.doi.org/10.1021/acsami.6b09772]

[17] Oerlemans C, Bult W, Bos M, Storm G, Nijsen JF, Hennink WE. Polymeric micelles in anticancer therapy: targeting, imaging and triggered release. Pharm Res 2010; 27(12): 2569-89.
[http://dx.doi.org/10.1007/s11095-010-0233-4] [PMID: 20725771]

[18] Zhang X, Huang Y, Li S. Nanomicellar carriers for targeted delivery of anticancer agents. Ther Deliv 2014; 5(1): 53-68.
[http://dx.doi.org/10.4155/tde.13.135] [PMID: 24341817]

[19] Moss JA. HIV/AIDS Review. Radiol Technol 2013; 84(3): 247-67.
[PMID: 23322863]

[20] Bartlett JG, Moore RD. Improving HIV therapy. Sci Am 1998; 279(1): 84-87, 89.
[http://dx.doi.org/10.1038/scientificamerican0798-84] [PMID: 9648300]

[21] Crabtree-Ramírez B, Villasís-Keever A, Galindo-Fraga A, del Río C, Sierra-Madero J. Effectiveness of highly active antiretroviral therapy (HAART) among HIV-infected patients in Mexico. AIDS Res Hum Retroviruses 2010; 26(4): 373-8.
[http://dx.doi.org/10.1089/aid.2009.0077] [PMID: 20377418]

[22] Jayant R, Nair M. Nanotechnology for the treatment of NeuroAIDS. J Nanomed Res 2016; 3(1): 00047.
[http://dx.doi.org/10.15406/jnmr.2016.03.00047]

[23] Rao KS, Ghorpade A, Labhasetwar V. Targeting anti-HIV drugs to the CNS. Expert Opin Drug Deliv 2009; 6(8): 771-84.

[http://dx.doi.org/10.1517/17425240903081705] [PMID: 19566446]

[24] Aggarwal BB, Van Kuiken ME, Iyer LH, Harikumar KB, Sung B. Molecular targets of nutraceuticals derived from dietary spices: potential role in suppression of inflammation and tumorigenesis. Exp Biol Med (Maywood) 2009; 234(8): 825-49. [http://dx.doi.org/10.3181/0902-MR-78] [PMID: 19491364]

[25] Acosta E. Bioavailability of nanoparticles in nutrient and nutraceutical delivery. Curr. Opin. Colloid Interface Sci. 2009; 14(1): 3-15. [http://dx.doi.org/10.1016/j.cocis.2008.01.002]

[26] Shaikh J, Ankola DD, Beniwal V, Singh D, Kumar MN. Nanoparticle encapsulation improves oral bioavailability of curcumin by at least 9-fold when compared to curcumin administered with piperine as absorption enhancer. Eur J Pharm Sci : Off J Eur Fed Pharm Sci 2009; 37(3-4): 223-30. [PMID: 19491009]

[27] Summerlin N, Soo E, Thakur S, Qu Z, Jambhrunkar S, Popat A. Resveratrol nanoformulations: challenges and opportunities. Int J Pharm 2015; 479(2): 282-90. [http://dx.doi.org/10.1016/j.ijpharm.2015.01.003] [PMID: 25572692]

[28] Rizvi SAA, Saleh AM. Applications of nanoparticle systems in drug delivery technology. Saudi Pharm J 2018; 26(1): 64-70. [http://dx.doi.org/10.1016/j.jsps.2017.10.012] [PMID: 29379334]

[29] Ventola CL. Progress in nanomedicine: approved and investigational nanodrugs. P & T: A peer-reviewed J Formulary Manag 2017; 42(12): 742-55. [PMID: 29234213]

[30] Tran S, DeGiovanni PJ, Piel B, Rai P. Cancer nanomedicine: a review of recent success in drug delivery. Clin Transl Med 2017; 6(1): 44. [http://dx.doi.org/10.1186/s40169-017-0175-0] [PMID: 29230567]

[31] Souery WN, Bishop CJ. Clinically advancing and promising polymer-based therapeutics. Acta Biomater 2018; 67: 1-20. [http://dx.doi.org/10.1016/j.actbio.2017.11.044] [PMID: 29246651]

[32] Fattal E, Hillaireau H, Mura S, Nicolas J, Tsapis N. Targeted delivery using biodegradable polymeric nanoparticles. In: Boston MA, Siepmann J, Siegel RA, Rathbone MJ, Eds. Fundamentals and Applications of Controlled Release Drug Delivery. US: Springer 2012; pp. 255-88. [http://dx.doi.org/10.1007/978-1-4614-0881-9_10]

[33] Yoo HS, Park TG. Biodegradable polymeric micelles composed of doxorubicin conjugated PLGA-PEG block copolymer. J Contr Rel 2001; 70(1-2): 63-70. [http://dx.doi.org/10.1016/S0168-3659(00)00340-0] [PMID: 11166408]

[34] Vu-Quang H, Vinding MS, Nielsen T, Ullisch MG, Nielsen NC, Kjems J. Theranostic tumor targeted nanoparticles combining drug delivery with dual near infrared and ^{19}F magnetic resonance imaging modalities. Nanomedicine (Lond) 2016; 12(7): 1873-84. [http://dx.doi.org/10.1016/j.nano.2016.04.010] [PMID: 27133191]

[35] Din FU, Aman W, Ullah I, *et al.* Effective use of nanocarriers as drug delivery systems for the treatment of selected tumors. Int J Nanomedicine 2017; 12: 7291-309. [http://dx.doi.org/10.2147/IJN.S146315] [PMID: 29042776]

[36] Tønnesen HH, Karlsen J. Alginate in drug delivery systems. Drug Dev Ind Pharm 2002; 28(6): 621-30. [http://dx.doi.org/10.1081/DDC-120003853] [PMID: 12149954]

[37] Patra JK, Das G, Fraceto LF, Campos EVR, Rodriguez-Torres MdP, Acosta-Torres LS, *et al.* Nano based drug delivery systems: recent developments and future prospects. J Nanobiotechnology 2018; 16(1): 71.

[38] Benny IS, Varadarajan G, Ponnusami V. Review on application of Xanthan gum in drug delivery. Int

J PharmTech Res 2014; 6(4): 1322-6.

[39] Meng LY, Wang B, Ma MG, Zhu JF. Cellulose-based nanocarriers as platforms for cancer therapy. Curr Pharm Des 2017; 23(35): 5292-300.
[PMID: 29086678]

[40] Allen TM, Cullis PR. Liposomal drug delivery systems: from concept to clinical applications. Adv Drug Deliv Rev 2013; 65(1): 36-48.
[http://dx.doi.org/10.1016/j.addr.2012.09.037] [PMID: 23036225]

[41] Immordino ML, Dosio F, Cattel L. Stealth liposomes: review of the basic science, rationale, and clinical applications, existing and potential. Int J Nanomedicine 2006; 1(3): 297-315.
[PMID: 17717971]

[42] Tomalia DA, Naylor AM, Goddard WA. Starburst dendrimers: molecular-level control of size, shape, surface chemistry, topology, and flexibility from atoms to macroscopic matter. Angewandte Chemie International Edition in English 1990; 29(2): 138-75.

[43] Duncan R, Izzo L. Dendrimer biocompatibility and toxicity. Adv Drug Deliv Rev 2005; 57(15): 2215-37.
[http://dx.doi.org/10.1016/j.addr.2005.09.019] [PMID: 16297497]

[44] Arora N, Thangavelu K, Karanikolos GN. Bimetallic nanoparticles for antimicrobial applications. Front Chem 2020; 8: 412.
[PMID: 32671014] [http://dx.doi.org/10.3389/fchem.2020.00412]

[45] Chen Z, Zhang A, Wang X, Zhu J, Fan Y, Yu H, *et al.* The advances of carbon nanotubes in cancer diagnostics and therapeutics. J Nanomater 2017; 2017: 1-13.
[http://dx.doi.org/10.1155/2017/3418932]

[46] Lay CL, Liu J, Liu Y. Functionalized carbon nanotubes for anticancer drug delivery. Expert Rev Med Devices 2011; 8(5): 561-6.
[http://dx.doi.org/10.1586/erd.11.34] [PMID: 22026621]

[47] Connor EE, Mwamuka J, Gole A, Murphy CJ, Wyatt MD. Gold nanoparticles are taken up by human cells but do not cause acute cytotoxicity. Small (Weinheim an der Bergstrasse, Germany) 2005; 1(3): 325-7.
[PMID: 17193451] [http://dx.doi.org/10.1002/smll.200400093]

[48] Shenoy D, Fu W, Li J, *et al.* Surface functionalization of gold nanoparticles using hetero-bifunctional poly(ethylene glycol) spacer for intracellular tracking and delivery. Int J Nanomedicine 2006; 1(1): 51-7.
[http://dx.doi.org/10.2147/nano.2006.1.1.51] [PMID: 16467923]

[49] Probst CE, Zrazhevskiy P, Bagalkot V, Gao X. Quantum dots as a platform for nanoparticle drug delivery vehicle design. Adv Drug Deliv Rev 2013; 65(5): 703-18.
[http://dx.doi.org/10.1016/j.addr.2012.09.036] [PMID: 23000745]

[50] Xu G, Zeng S, Zhang B, Swihart MT, Yong K-T, Prasad PN. New generation cadmium-free quantum dots for biophotonics and nanomedicine. Chem Rev 2016; 116(19): 12234-327.
[http://dx.doi.org/10.1021/acs.chemrev.6b00290] [PMID: 27657177]

[51] Zheng FF, Zhang PH, Xi Y, Chen JJ, Li LL, Zhu JJ. Aptamer/graphene quantum dots nanocomposite capped fluorescent mesoporous silica nanoparticles for intracellular drug delivery and real-time monitoring of drug release. Anal Chem 2015; 87(23): 11739-45.
[http://dx.doi.org/10.1021/acs.analchem.5b03131] [PMID: 26524192]

[52] Huang C-L, Huang C-C, Mai F-D, Yen C-L, Tzing S-H, Hsieh H-T, *et al.* Application of paramagnetic graphene quantum dots as a platform for simultaneous dual-modality bioimaging and tumor-targeted drug delivery. J Mater Chem B 2015; 3(4): 651-4.
[PMID: 32262348]

[53] Palanisamy S, Wang Y-M. Superparamagnetic iron oxide nanoparticulate system: synthesis, targeting,

drug delivery and therapy in cancer. Dalton Trans 2019; 48(26): 9490-515.
[http://dx.doi.org/10.1039/C9DT00459A] [PMID: 31211303]

[54] Xu ZP, Zeng QH, Lu GQ, Yu AB. Inorganic nanoparticles as carriers for efficient cellular delivery. Chem Engin Sci 2006; 61(3): 1027-40.
[http://dx.doi.org/10.1016/j.ces.2005.06.019]

[55] Wahajuddin AS, Arora S. Superparamagnetic iron oxide nanoparticles: magnetic nanoplatforms as drug carriers. Int J Nanomedicine 2012; 7: 3445-71.
[http://dx.doi.org/10.2147/IJN.S30320] [PMID: 22848170]

[56] Kukowska-Latallo JF, Bielinska AU, Johnson J, Spindler R, Tomalia DA, Baker JR Jr. Efficient transfer of genetic material into mammalian cells using Starburst polyamidoamine dendrimers. Proc Natl Acad Sci USA 1996; 93(10): 4897-902.
[http://dx.doi.org/10.1073/pnas.93.10.4897] [PMID: 8643500]

[57] Lin W, Huang YW, Zhou XD, Ma Y. In vitro toxicity of silica nanoparticles in human lung cancer cells. Toxicol Appl Pharmacol 2006; 217(3): 252-9.
[http://dx.doi.org/10.1016/j.taap.2006.10.004] [PMID: 17112558]

[58] Kim IY, Joachim E, Choi H, Kim K. Toxicity of silica nanoparticles depends on size, dose, and cell type. Nanomedicine (Lond) 2015; 11(6): 1407-16.
[http://dx.doi.org/10.1016/j.nano.2015.03.004] [PMID: 25819884]

[59] Hu JJ, Liu LH, Li ZY, Zhuo RX, Zhang XZ. MMP-responsive theranostic nanoplatform based on mesoporous silica nanoparticles for tumor imaging and targeted drug delivery. J Mater Chem B 2016; 4(11): 1932-40.
[http://dx.doi.org/10.1039/C5TB02490K] [PMID: 32263070]

[60] Lombardo D, Kiselev MA, Caccamo MT. Smart nanoparticles for drug delivery application: development of versatile nanocarrier platforms in biotechnology and nanomedicine. J Nanomat 2019; 3702518.

CHAPTER 5

Nanoparticle-DNA Conjugate: The Treatment and Diagnostic Option for Future Cure of Diseases

Abstract: Integrated DNA in nanoparticles show unique and augmented properties due to their synergistic activity on the biological system. Their capabilities are attracting the attention of researchers for their wide variety of applications in diagnostics, therapeutics, theranostics, biosensing, labeling, imaging, *etc.* In this study, we discuss these nanohybrids and their area of application. DNA incorporated within these nanoparticles helps in gene delivery to the targeted tissue. Sometimes, DNA aptamers can recognize specific target sequence by complementarity. They can target specific cell/tissue/organ to deliver their payload to that target site. However, it is clear that there are more things to be revealed in the application of nanoparticles in the biological system. The unique properties of nanomaterial have more to offer in this field of nanotechnology.

Keywords: Biosensing, Carbon nanotube, Colorimetic detection, Deoxyribonucleic acid, Electrochemical detection, Fluorescence detection, Gene delivery, Gene therapy, Gold nanoparticle, Imaging, Labeling, Microarray, Nanobiotechnology, Nanocrystal, Nanohybrid, Nanomaterial, Nanoparticle, Plasmonic application, Silver nanoparticle, Theranostic.

INTRODUCTION

Nanotechnology in its manifestation is developing new technologies, new materials, new functionality and new therapeutic interventions for a wide variety of disease conditions. In its first step, nanotechnology developed a variety of nanomaterials or nanocrystals or nanoparticles with a large variation of optical, magnetic, mechanical, physical and chemical properties. With the synthesis of nanoparticles, the parameters may be changed and modified so that they can demonstrate a wide variety of size, shape, surface to volume ratio that makes them unique. These nanomaterials find a variety of applications in non-biological fields such as improved data storage, energy harvesting in solar cells, optical displays, chemical catalysis and for purification purposes.

From these wide varieties of nanoparticles, deoxyribonucleic acid (DNA) is found to have a potential application in the biomedical field . Within the last decade,

Rituparna Acharya

DNA and other nucleic acids are demonstrating significant contribution in the field of diagnostics, theranostics and gene therapy. These macromolecules are mainly exploited due to their ability to recognize genomic sequences, complementarity and hybridization ability by using them as probes. The other utility of DNA is in the form of aptamers that are highly specific for particular DNA sequence and can target cell surface markers as well.

The ongoing research on nanotechnology is focused on the production of hybrid materials that can have diagnostic and therapeutic applications in the biomedical field. These nanomaterials have value-added application in the field of bionanotechnology using their theranostic properties. This property enables diagnosis and therapeutic applications at the same time by targeted delivery of nanomaterial with its hybrid structure to the target tissue with specific interest. The biological macromolecules such as peptide, antibodies or aptamers can recognize specific target tissue/organ/cell while the nanoparticle will be the host that will also carry the payload of drugs or nucleic acids.

Moreover, encapsulated nanoparticles help to overcome many disadvantages of the nanoparticles that are used in bare form. The main advantage of encapsulated nanoparticles is to overcome the toxic effect of the bare form. Nanoparticles may also encapsulate DNA and other biological macromolecules to have their therapeutic and diagnostic applications.

Our focus is to identify the unique properties of the nanoparticles when hybridized with DNA in the biomedical field. We are intended to identify the area of application of nanoparticles when synergistic with DNA in bionanotechnology. This study has direct interest in gene therapy/gene silencing/and gene delivery that has commercial and research interest. Rather than focusing on every combination of nanoparticle-DNA conjugate, we are intended to discuss those hybrids that have potential application in the biomedical area. This study is divided into various types of potential nanoparticles than their hybrids of DNA and their applications in the field of nanobiotechnology. In the previous chapters we have already discussed the nanoparticle synthesis method but in this chapter, we only focus on specific important nanoparticles that have significant applications in the biomedical field.

DNA-NANOPARTICLE CONJUGATES IN NANOMEDICINE

DNAs are the carrier of genetic information in our body from generation to generation. It is a double helix structure that makes it double-stranded DNA (dsDNA). Polymerization of nucleotides makes each DNA strand unite. Each nucleotide comprises 3 components i. e., one sugar molecule, one phosphodiester group and one nitrogenous base. DNA has four types of nitrogenous bases or nucleo bases *i.e.,* adenine, guanine, cytosine and thymine. Adenine and guanine are purine while cytosine and thymine are pyrimidine bases. Adenine binds with thymine by 2 hydrogen bonds and cytosine binds with guanine by 3 hydrogen bonds.

Single DNA and nanoparticle can bind with each other by specific and nonspecific bindings. DNA can covalently bind on the surface of the nanoparticle through anchor groups, such as –OH,–SH, $-NH_2$ or –COOH. The nonspecific bindings can be achieved by non-covalent interaction *via* simple adsorption. The understanding of these bindings in the molecular is necessary in order to monitor the conjugate at the site of application.

DNA-Gold Nanoparticle Conjugate

Goldnanoparticles are highly studied area of research in today's world. It has a wide area of application that includes imaging, sensing, catalysis, diagnostics, therapeutics and drug delivery etc [1 - 3].

Binding Between DNA and Gold Nanoparticle

Single stranded DNA binds better than the double stranded DNA with the gold nanoparticle. It has been believed that double stranded DNA as they are negatively charged, experience repulsion from the gold nanoparticle that comprises of negatively charged surface [4]. On the other hand single stranded DNAs are flexible and easily wraps around the gold nanoparticle. However, there are several drawbacks of using single stranded DNA such as the binding between the DNA and gold nanoparticle becomes weak in high temperature (50°C) and also in room temperature single stranded DNA produces hairpin structure. Moreover, long single stranded DNAs are not found to bind with the gold nanoparticle [5]. It can be stated that the binding affinity is largely dependent on the particle size.

Application of DNA-Gold Nanoconjugate in Nucleic Acid Detection

ssDNA and dsDNA adsorption on the surface of gold nanoparticle is different. Using this principle Li et. al., demonstrated a hybridization assay for the detection of untagged oligonucleotides at a detection level as low as 4.3nm. The assay is simple, highly sensitive and don't need expensive device to estimate the specific oligonucleotides [6].

Other than this *in vitro* assay, DNA-gold nanoconjugate is also utilized for the estimation of specific mRNA within the cell. The Mirkin group in this method utilized gold nanoparticle with thiolated DNA with specific sequence for the detection of mRNA. In the presence of specific mRNA fluorescent signals are detected [7].

Application of DNA-Gold Nanoparticle for Colorimetric Detection of Miscellaneous Analytes

Cancer cells may be detected by colorimetric detection as well [8]. DNA in this method is thiol-functionalized aptamer that are targeted to cancer cells. Gold nanoparticles can carry multiple numbers of aptamers that binds on the cancer cells and changes the color from red to purple.

Many other forms of aptamer conjugated with gold nanoparticles may be used for biomedical detection purposes. These applications are the detection of thrombin *i.e.*, most important molecule for blood coagulation [9]. Similar detection method can also be employed for lysozyme which is associated with diseases such as leukemia and tuberculosis [10]. Some simple modification of aptamer-gold nanoconjugate can also determine the ATP and cocaine that makes them versatile recognition element [11].

Mirkin's group have demonstrated that DNA-gold nanoconjugate may bind with antitumor agents like amsacrine, ellipticine and daunorubicin [12]. This conjugate can also be used for the detection of toxic metal ions such as Hg^{2+} and Pb^{2+} [13 - 16]. Huang *et al.* developed nanoconjugate that is used as a sensor for the detection of plateletderived growth factor (PDGF) [17].

Application of DNA-Gold Nanoconjugate for Gene And Drug Delivery

Gold nanoparticles are used for therapeutic purposes from ancient time [18]. They are highly applicable for gene therapy and drug delivery as they biocompatible, less toxic, and stable in blood and intracellular environment [19]. The double stranded DNA is found to be highly stable in the blood against any enzymatic degradation. Oligonucleotide functionalized gold nanoparticle may also be covalently linked with the anticancer drugs that may be delivered on the target site. Plasmid encoding β-galactoside, enhanced green fluorescent proteins (eGFP) *etc.* are conjugated with gold nanoparticles are used in several cell lines and observed that they are working within the cells [20, 21].

DNA-Silver Conjugate Nanoparticle

In respect to gold nanoparticles, silver nanoparticles are far better in their diagnostic applications. The reason behind this is because the bonding between silver nanoparticle and DNA is much weaker than gold nanoparticle and DNA bonding. To increase the strength in the bonding multithiol moieties are incorporated within the DNA structure.

Plasmonic Application of DNA-Silver Nanoconjugate

Silver nanoparticles are utilized for biosensing in dark field microscopy. Single stranded DNA was utilized with biotin and streptavidin to identify the distance between two nanospheres. Single stranded DNA probes are used for this purpose with biotin on one end and streptavidin on the other. The hybridized DNA demonstrates significant blue shift at plasmonic resonance.

DNA-Magnetic Nanoparticle

Magnetic nanoparticles are mainly maghemite (γ-Fe_3O_4) and magnetite(Fe_3O_4) have demonstrated their application in diverse areas including catalysis, labeling,sensing,magnetic resonance imaging (MRI) in the area of biomedical field [22 - 27].

Gene Therapy

Magnetic nanoparticles are excellent gene delivery vehicle just only by adsorbing the DNA on to its surface. DNA vector by the help of magnetic nanoparticle have reduced dosage and transfection time in several cell lines such as lung epithelial cells and blood vascular endothelial cells *etc.* A high DNA surface density produces some unique characteristics such as low enzymatic degradation of the DNA and increased cellular uptake [28]. High cellular uptake was demonstrated in Hela cells without the presence of transfection reagent [29].

Fluorescence Detection Method

Novel nanoparticle based fluorescence detection was determined by using magnetic nanoparticles. Sandwich hybridization strategy was followed using DNA. Specific target DNA was first hybridized using oligonucleotide immobilized with magnetic nanoparticle. Then it is hybridized with oligonucleotide probe immobilized on gold nanoparticle. Amplified DNA signals are detected using chip based fluorescence detector. This system can be employed for the detection of DNA and immunoassay [30].

DNA-Platinum and Palladium Nanoparticles

Impressive progress has been demonstrated from last decade on the synthesis of platinum nanoparticle of various size and shapes [31 - 33]. The catalytic efficiency of this nanoparticle largely depends upon the size, shape, surface ligand and solvent [34, 35].

Electrochemical Detection

Willner group demonstrated that DNA modified platinum nanoparticle may detect DNA and thrombin electrochemically. For detecting DNA oligonucleotides are immobilized on platinum nanoparticle and gold electrode. In the presence of target DNA the platinum nanoparticle attaches itself on gold electrode and produces a catalytic reaction that can be noticed on cyclic voltammeter. Similarly thrombin protein is also detected using DNA-platinum nanoconjugate [36].

DNA Detection in Chip Based Microarrays

Wang and coworkers used amine-modified DNA to conjugate with palladium nanoparticle synthesized inaqueous media. The resultant nanoconjugate demonstrated stability in saline solution and was further employed for the detection of DNA in chip based microarray method. The target DNA is detected in this method as the complementary DNA conjugated with palladium was captured by the target DNA and in subsequent steps the change is color was found [37].

DNA-Quantum Dots Nanoconjugate

Quantum dot-functionalized DNA templates have several biological applications. DNA-quantum dot conjugate have broadly few applications in biosensing and therapeutics that will be discussed over here:

Biosensing Application

DNA-quantum dot nanoconjugates are widely used for the detection of DNA, RNA, mRNA and miRNA and several other molecular ligands. FRET based biosensing device was fabricated using DNA-quantum dot nanoconjugates [38, 39]. Another application method is fluorescence in situ hybridization (FISH) that also applies the same nanoconjugate [40, 41]. The DNA-quantum dot-fluorophore-FRET method are found to be more robust, sensitive and highly quantitative in their application. These biosensing assays has definitely improved the reliability of the detection and improved the current state of art.

Gene Delivery and Therapeutics

The DNA-quantum dot nanoconjugates are found to be highly reasonable for the delivery of gene and therapeutics because of mainly two reasons. First of all quantum dot nanoparticles have a high surface to volume ratio that makes them highly competent of carrying large payloads. Secondly, they are highly stable that enable them to stay within the cell for longer period of time [42].

Enhanced green fluorescent protein (EFGP) was used loaded in the DNA plasmid and that was conjugated with quantum dot nanoparticle demonstrated the nanoconjugate as an ideal one for gene delivery [43]. Another class of therapeutic intervention by quantum dot was using DNA as siRNA mediated gene silencing [44, 45].

DNA-Carbon Nanotubes

DNA-carbon nanotube has wide range of application in the field of biosensor, biological transporter [46], fiber for artificial muscle [47] and bioelectrodes for fuel cells [48]. In the last few years the publications of the scientific application of these hybrids has increased exponentially. The application of these nanohybrides is discussed in detail in the following sections:

Chemical Biosensors

DNA-wrapped carbon nanotube are used for the detection of various substrates such as glucose, peroxide, dopamine, pesticides [49], vapor [50], protein [51], ions *etc.* For the detection of dopamine DNA-wrapped carbon nanotubes are deposited on the glass substrate [52]. Change in the near infra-red luminous intensity of the glucose-DNA-single walled carbon nanotube in presence of glucose helps the detection of it at micro molar concentration [53]. Peroxide was detected in the presence of hemoglobin by DNA-single walled carbon nanotube [54]. Based on DNA-carbon nanotube, field effect transistor (FET) device detects five different odors that have low recovery time and excellent reproducibility [55]. DNA-wrapped single walled carbon nanotube may act as a detection device for wide range of ions by a shift in band gap in the emission and absorption spectra [56].

Detection of Nucleic Acid Sequence

DNA-wrapped carbon nanotube may detect the nucleic acid with specific sequence by the help of Field effect transistors (FETs). Hwang and coworkers used DNA-single walled carbon nanotube for the detection of particular DNA from the complex genome [57].

Biological Transporters

Various publications have established that DNA-wrapped carbon nanotube is more stable structure than bare DNA within the cell. DNA bound within single walled carbon nanotubes is safe from DNAse enzymes that are present in the blood and have the property to digest the bare DNA. These protected DNA probes have high stability and delivery capacity against bare DNA probes [58].

DNA-Chitosan Nanoparticle

Chitosan-DNA nanoconjugate is prepared using a complex coacervation process. Important parameters for synthesis are detected by Mao *et al.* The parameters are pH, concentration of DNA and chitosan and also the molecular weight.

Gene Therapy

DNA within the chitosan nanoparticles is partially protected from the enzymes that degrade the DNA in the blood. The transfection efficiency of the nanoconjugate is highly cell-specific. PEGylated nanoparticle is slow in the clearance through kidney than unmodified nanoparticle when administered intravenously (Fig. **1**) [59].

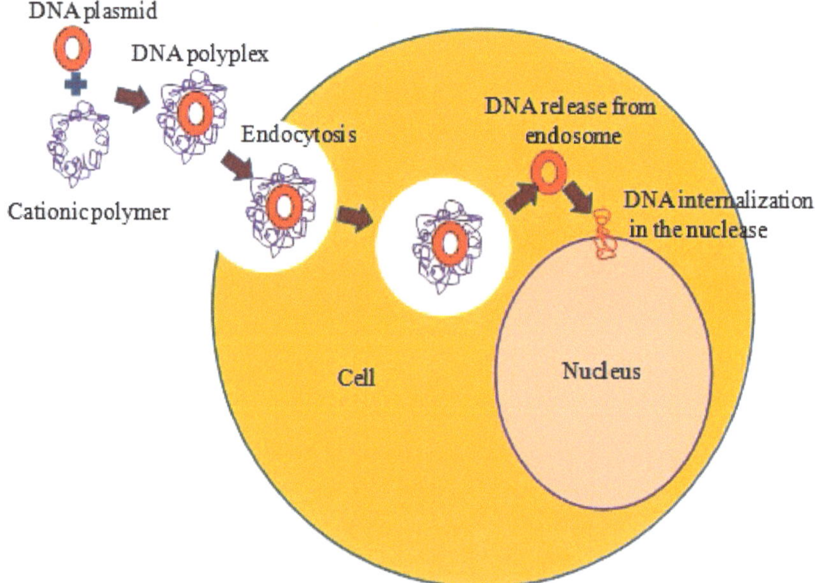

Fig. (1). DNA cellular internalization using cationic polymer.

CONCLUSION

The above study has covered the application areas of nanoparticles in conjugation with DNA. The partnership of these materials is steadily growing along with the new areas of application. New types of materials in conjugation with varied types of DNA sequences are being explored in everyday research all over the world. The interaction between multi-active materials with DNA has a strong potential application in diverse fields. Interaction of new materials with DNA is giving rise to new biosensing properties that may be exploited in biomedical engineering.

From the above-mentioned areas of application, we may get a roadmap for future areas of biosensing and gene therapy. New capabilities will be revealed as the application will grow in their complexity and sophistication. We may expect more avenues will be addressed by continuous research in nanomaterials and biological macromolecules [60, 61]. Nanomachines and nanodevices will develop in near future to diagnose disease conditions as portable diagnostic applications. Along with the nanoparticles, DNA will also demonstrate gene therapy and diagnostic biosensing applications. The above study is intended to provide a roadmap for future applicability of new nanomaterials and biological particles.

REFERENCES

[1] Boisselier E, Astruc D. Gold nanoparticles in nanomedicine: preparations, imaging, diagnostics, therapies and toxicity. Chem Soc Rev 2009; 38(6): 1759-82. [http://dx.doi.org/10.1039/b806051g] [PMID: 19587967]

[2] Dreaden EC, Alkilany AM, Huang X, Murphy CJ, El-Sayed MA. The golden age: gold nanoparticles for biomedicine. Chem Soc Rev 2012; 41(7): 2740-79. [http://dx.doi.org/10.1039/C1CS15237H] [PMID: 22109657]

[3] Huang X, Jain PK, El-Sayed IH, El-Sayed MA. Gold nanoparticles: interesting optical properties and recent applications in cancer diagnostics and therapy. Nanomedicine (Lond) 2007; 2(5): 681-93. [http://dx.doi.org/10.2217/17435889.2.5.681] [PMID: 17976030]

[4] Gaylord B, Heeger A, Bazan G. DNA detection using water-soluble conjugated polymers and peptide nucleic acid probes. Proc Nat Acad Sci USA. 99(17): 10954-57. [http://dx.doi.org/10.1073/pnas.162375999]

[5] Zanchet D, Micheel C, Parak W, Gerion D, Alivisatos A. Electrophoretic isolation of discrete au nanocrystal/dna conjugates. Nano Lett 2000; 1(1): 32-5.

[6] Li H, Rothberg L. Colorimetric detection of DNA sequences based on electrostatic interactions with unmodified gold nanoparticles. Proc Natl Acad Sci USA 2004; 101(39): 14036-9. [http://dx.doi.org/10.1073/pnas.0406115101] [PMID: 15381774]

[7] Seferos DS, Giljohann DA, Hill HD, Prigodich AE, Mirkin CA. Nano-Flares: Probes for transfection and mrna detection in living cells. J Am Chem Soc 2007; 129(50): 15477-9.

[8] Medley CD, Smith JE, Tang Z, Wu Y, Bamrungsap S, Tan W. Gold nanoparticle-based colorimetric assay for the direct detection of cancerous cells. Anal Chem 2008; 80(4): 1067-72. [http://dx.doi.org/10.1021/ac702037y] [PMID: 18198894]

[9] Pavlov V, Xiao Y, Shlyahovsky B, Willner I. Aptamer-functionalized au nanoparticles for the amplified optical detection of thrombin. J Am Chem Soc 2004; 126(38): 11768-9. [http://dx.doi.org/10.1021/ja046970u]

[10] Wang X, Xu Y, Chen Y, Li L, Liu F, Li N. he gold-nanoparticle-based surface plasmon resonance light scattering and visual DNA aptasensor for lysozyme. Anal Bioanal Chem 2011; 400(7): 2085-91. [http://dx.doi.org/10.1007/s00216-011-4943-1] [PMID: 21461986]

[11] Liu J, Lu Y. Fast colorimetric sensing of adenosine and cocaine based on a general sensor design involving aptamers and nanoparticles. Angew Chem Int Ed Engl 2005; 45(1): 90-4. [http://dx.doi.org/10.1002/anie.200502589] [PMID: 16292781]

[12] Han MS, Lytton-Jean AK, Oh BK, Heo J, Mirkin CA. Colorimetric screening of DNA-binding molecules with gold nanoparticle probes. Angew Chem Int Ed Engl 2006; 45(11): 1807-10. [http://dx.doi.org/10.1002/anie.200504277] [PMID: 16482507]

[13] Liu CW, Hsieh YT, Huang CC, Lin ZH, Chang HT. Detection of mercury(II) based on Hg^{2+} -DNA complexes inducing the aggregation of gold nanoparticles. Chem Commun (Cambridge, England) 2008; 21(19): 2242-4.
[PMID: 18463753]

[14] Li D, Wieckowska A, Willner I. Optical analysis of Hg^{2+} ions by oligonucleotide-gold-nanoparticle hybrids and DNA-based machines. Angew Chem Int Ed Engl 2008; 47(21): 3927-31.
[http://dx.doi.org/10.1002/anie.200705991] [PMID: 18404745]

[15] Wang H, Wang Y, Jin J, Yang R. Gold nanoparticle-based colorimetric and "turn-On" fluorescent probe for mercury(II) ions in aqueous solution. Anal Chem 2008; 80(23): 9021-8.

[16] Liu J, Lu Y. A colorimetric lead biosensor using DNAzyme-Directed assembly of gold nanoparticles. J Am Chem Soc 2003; 125(22): 6642-3.
[http://dx.doi.org/10.1021/ja034775u]

[17] Huang CC, Chiu SH, Huang YF, Chang HT. Aptamer-functionalized gold nanoparticles for turn-on light switch detection of platelet-derived growth factor. Anal Chem 2007; 79(13): 4798-804.
[http://dx.doi.org/10.1021/ac0707075] [PMID: 17530743]

[18] Jeong EH, Jung G, Hong CA, Lee H. Gold nanoparticle (AuNP)-based drug delivery and molecular imaging for biomedical applications. Arch Pharm Res 2014; 37(1): 53-9.
[http://dx.doi.org/10.1007/s12272-013-0273-5] [PMID: 24214174]

[19] Seferos DS, Prigodich AE, Giljohann DA, Patel PC, Mirkin CA. Polyvalent DNA nanoparticle conjugates stabilize nucleic acids. Nano Lett 2009; 9(1): 308-11.
[http://dx.doi.org/10.1021/nl802958f] [PMID: 19099465]

[20] Sandhu KK, McIntosh CM, Simard JM, Smith SW, Rotello VM. Gold nanoparticle-mediated transfection of mammalian cells. Bioconjug Chem 2002; 13(1): 3-6.
[http://dx.doi.org/10.1021/bc015545c] [PMID: 11792172]

[21] Yang W. Nucleases: diversity of structure, function and mechanism. Q Rev Biophys 2011; 44(1): 1-93.
[http://dx.doi.org/10.1017/S0033583510000181] [PMID: 20854710]

[22] Fang C, Zhang M. Multifunctional magnetic nanoparticles for medical imaging applications. J Mater Chem 2009; 19(35): 6258-66.
[http://dx.doi.org/10.1039/b902182e] [PMID: 20593005]

[23] Lu AH, Salabas EL, Schüth F. Magnetic nanoparticles: synthesis, protection, functionalization, and application. Angew Chem Int Ed Engl 2007; 46(8): 1222-44.
[http://dx.doi.org/10.1002/anie.200602866] [PMID: 17278160]

[24] Pankhurst QA, Connolly J, Jones SK, Dobson J. Applications of magnetic nanoparticles in biomedicine. J Phys D Appl Phys 2003; 36(13): 591-626.
[http://dx.doi.org/10.1088/0022-3727/36/13/201]

[25] Abu-Reziq R, Alper H, Wang D, Post ML. Metal supported on dendronized magnetic nanoparticles: Highly selective hydroformylation catalysts. J Am Chem Soc 2006; 128(15): 5279-82.

[26] Frey NA, Peng S, Cheng K, Sun S. Magnetic nanoparticles: synthesis, functionalization, and applications in bioimaging and magnetic energy storage. Chem Soc Rev 2009; 38(9): 2532-42.
[http://dx.doi.org/10.1039/b815548h] [PMID: 19690734]

[27] Sun X, Huang Y, Nikles D. FePt and CoPt Magnetic Nanoparticles Film for Future High Density Data Storage Media. ChemInform 2005; 12/27: 36.
[http://dx.doi.org/10.1002/chin.200552214]

[28] Sapsford KE, Algar WR, Berti L, *et al.* Functionalizing nanoparticles with biological molecules: developing chemistries that facilitate nanotechnology. Chem Rev 2013; 113(3): 1904-2074.

[http://dx.doi.org/10.1021/cr300143v] [PMID: 23432378]

[29] Lan X, Chen Z, Dai G, Lu X, Ni W, Wang Q. Bifacial DNA origami-directed discrete, three-dimensional, anisotropic plasmonic nanoarchitectures with tailored optical chirality. J Am Chem Soc 2013; 135(31): 11441-4.

[30] Nie LB, Wang XL, Li S, Chen H. Amplification of fluorescence detection of DNA based on magnetic separation. Int J Japan Soc Anal Chem 2009; 25(11): 1327-31. [http://dx.doi.org/10.2116/analsci.25.1327] [PMID: 19907090]

[31] Wang C, Daimon H, Onodera T, Koda T, Sun S. A general approach to the size- and shape-controlled synthesis of platinum nanoparticles and their catalytic reduction of oxygen. Angew Chem Int Ed Engl 2008; 47(19): 3588-91. [http://dx.doi.org/10.1002/anie.200800073] [PMID: 18399516]

[32] Ahmadi TS, Wang ZL, Green TC, Henglein A, El-Sayed MA. Shape-Controlled Synthesis of Colloidal Platinum Nanoparticles. Science 1996; 272(5270): 1924-6. [http://dx.doi.org/10.1126/science.272.5270.1924] [PMID: 8662492]

[33] Long NV, Chien N, Hayakawa T, Hirata H, Lakshminarayana G, Nogami M. The synthesis and characterization of platinum nanoparticles: A method of controlling the size and morphology. Nanotechnology 2010; 21(3): 035605.

[34] Ye H, Crooks JA, Crooks RM. Effect of particle size on the kinetics of the electrocatalytic oxygen reduction reaction catalyzed by Pt dendrimer-encapsulated nanoparticles. Langmuir 2007; 23(23): 11901-6. [http://dx.doi.org/10.1021/la702297m]

[35] Narayanan R, El-Sayed MA. Effect of nanocatalysis in colloidal solution on the tetrahedral and cubic nanoparticle shape: electron-transfer reaction catalyzed by platinum nanoparticles. J Phys Chem B 2004; 108(18): 5726-33.

[36] Polsky R, Gill R, Kaganovsky L, Willner I. Nucleic acid-functionalized Pt nanoparticles: Catalytic labels for the amplified electrochemical detection of biomolecules. Anal Chem 2006; 78(7): 2268-71. [http://dx.doi.org/10.1021/ac0519864] [PMID: 16579607]

[37] Wang Z, Li H, Zhen S, He N. Preparation of carboxyl group-modified palladium nanoparticles in an aqueous solution and their conjugation with DNA. Nanoscale 2012; 4(11): 3536-42. [http://dx.doi.org/10.1039/c2nr30649b] [PMID: 22543815]

[38] Dubertret B. Quantum dots: DNA detectives. Nat Mater 2005; 4(11): 797-8. [http://dx.doi.org/10.1038/nmat1520] [PMID: 16379066]

[39] Algar WR, Krull UJ. Towards multi-colour strategies for the detection of oligonucleotide hybridization using quantum dots as energy donors in fluorescence resonance energy transfer (FRET). Anal Chim Acta 2007; 581(2): 193-201. [http://dx.doi.org/10.1016/j.aca.2006.08.026] [PMID: 17386444]

[40] Bentolila LA, Weiss S. Single-step multicolor fluorescence in situ hybridization using semiconductor quantum dot-DNA conjugates. Cell Biochem Biophys 2006; 45(1): 59-70. [http://dx.doi.org/10.1385/CBB:45:1:59] [PMID: 16679564]

[41] Xiao Y, Barker PE. Semiconductor nanocrystal probes for human metaphase chromosomes. Nucleic Acids Res 2004; 32(3): e28. [http://dx.doi.org/10.1093/nar/gnh024] [PMID: 14960711]

[42] Banerjee A, Pons T, Lequeux N, Dubertret B. Quantum dots-DNA bioconjugates: synthesis to applications. Interface Focus 2016; 6(6): 20160064. [http://dx.doi.org/10.1098/rsfs.2016.0064] [PMID: 27920898]

[43] Wu Y, Eisele K, Doroshenko M, Algara-Siller G, Kaiser U, Koynov K, *et al.* A quantum dot photoswitch for DNA detection, gene transfection, and live-cell imaging. Small (Weinheim an der

Bergstrasse, Germany) 2012; 8(22): 3465-75.
[http://dx.doi.org/10.1002/smll.201200409] [PMID: 22915540]

[44] Derfus AM, Chen AA, Min DH, Ruoslahti E, Bhatia SN. Targeted quantum dot conjugates for siRNA delivery. Bioconjug Chem 2007; 18(5): 1391-6.
[http://dx.doi.org/10.1021/bc060367e] [PMID: 17630789]

[45] Qi L, Gao X. Quantum dot-amphipol nanocomplex for intracellular delivery and real-time imaging of siRNA. ACS Nano 2008; 2(7): 1403-10.
[http://dx.doi.org/10.1021/nn800280r] [PMID: 19206308]

[46] Sánchez-Pomales G, Santiago-Rodríguez L, Cabrera CR. DNA-functionalized carbon nanotubes for biosensing applications. J Nanosci Nanotechnol 2009; 9(4): 2175-88.
[http://dx.doi.org/10.1166/jnn.2009.SE47] [PMID: 19437957]

[47] Shin S, Lee CK, So IS, Jeon JH, Kang T, Kee CW, *et al.* DNA-wrapped single-walled carbon nanotube hybrid fibers for supercapacitors and artificial muscles. Adv Mater 2008; 20(3): 466-70.
[http://dx.doi.org/10.1002/adma.200701102]

[48] Lee JY, Shin HY, Kang SW, Park C, Kim SW. Use of bioelectrode containing DNA-wrapped single-walled carbon nanotubes for enzyme-based biofuel cell. J. Power Sources 2010; 195(3): 750-5.

[49] Viswanathan S, Radecka H, Radecki J. Electrochemical biosensor for pesticides based on acetylcholinesterase immobilized on polyaniline deposited on vertically assembled carbon nanotubes wrapped with ssDNA. Biosens Bioelectron 2009; 24(9): 2772-7.
[http://dx.doi.org/10.1016/j.bios.2009.01.044]

[50] Staii C, Johnson AT Jr, Chen M, Gelperin A. DNA-decorated carbon nanotubes for chemical sensing. Nano Lett 2005; 5(9): 1774-8.
[http://dx.doi.org/10.1021/nl051261f] [PMID: 16159222]

[51] Wu Z, Zhen Z, Jiang JH, Shen GL, Yu RQ. Terminal protection of small-molecule-linked DNA for sensitive electrochemical detection of protein binding via selective carbon nanotube assembly. J Am Chem Soc 2009; 131(34): 12325-32.
[http://dx.doi.org/10.1021/ja9038054] [PMID: 19655753]

[52] Ma Y, Ali SR, Dodoo AS, He H. Enhanced sensitivity for biosensors: multiple functions of DNA-wrapped single-walled carbon nanotubes in self-doped polyaniline nanocomposites. J Phys Chem B 2006; 110(33): 16359-65.
[http://dx.doi.org/10.1021/jp0614897] [PMID: 16913764]

[53] Karachevtsev VA, Glamazda AY, Leontiev VS, Lytvyn OS, Dettlaff-Weglikowska U. Glucose sensing based on NIR fluorescence of DNA-wrapped single-walled carbon nanotubes. Chem Phys Lett 2007; 435(1): 104-8.

[54] Liang Z, Lao R, Wang J, Liu Y, Wang L, Huang Q, *et al.* Solubilization of single-walled carbon nanotubes with single-stranded dna generated from asymmetric PCR. Int J Mol Sci 2007; 8(7): 705-13.
[http://dx.doi.org/10.3390/i8070705] [PMID: PMC3716441]

[55] Poonam P, Deo N. Current correlation functions for chemical sensors based on DNA decorated carbon nanotube. Sens Actuators, B 2008; 135(1): 327-35.
[http://dx.doi.org/10.1016/j.snb.2008.09.003]

[56] Heller DA, Jeng ES, Yeung T-K, *et al.* Optical detection of DNA conformational polymorphism on single-walled carbon nanotubes. Science 2006; 311(5760): 508-11.
[http://dx.doi.org/10.1126/science.1120792] [PMID: 16439657]

[57] Hwang ES, Cao C, Hong S, *et al.* The DNA hybridization assay using single-walled carbon nanotubes as ultrasensitive, long-term optical labels. Nanotechnology 2006; 17(14): 3442-5.
[http://dx.doi.org/10.1088/0957-4484/17/14/016] [PMID: 19661588]

[58] Wu Y, Phillips JA, Liu H, Yang R, Tan W. Carbon nanotubes protect DNA strands during cellular delivery. ACS Nano 2008; 2(10): 2023-8.

[http://dx.doi.org/10.1021/nn800325a] [PMID: 19206447]

[59] Mao HQ, Roy K, Troung-Le VL, Janes KA, Lin KY, Wang Y, *et al.* Chitosan-DNA nanoparticles as gene carriers: synthesis, characterization and transfection efficiency. J Control Rel Soc 2001; 70(3): 399-421.
[http://dx.doi.org/10.1016/S0168-3659(00)00361-8] [PMID: 11182210]

[60] Breger J, Delehanty JB, Medintz IL. Continuing progress toward controlled intracellular delivery of semiconductor quantum dots. Wiley Interdiscip Rev Nanomed Nanobiotechnol 2015; 7(2). 131-51.
[http://dx.doi.org/10.1002/wnan.1281] [PMID: 25154379]

[61] Field LD, Delehanty JB, Chen Y, Medintz IL. Peptides for specifically targeting nanoparticles to cellular organelles: quo vadis? Acc Chem Res 2015; 48(5): 1380-90.
[http://dx.doi.org/10.1021/ar500449v] [PMID: 25853734]

CHAPTER 6

Nanoparticle Conjugated with siRNA for Treatment of Different Types of Disease Conditions

Abstract: Gene silencing is a mechanism by which several protein expressions may be controlled in eukaryotes. Since its invention, many studies have been performed for its diagnostic and therapeutic intervention. siRNAs have created special attention for the treatment of incurable and difficult disease conditions. However, there are many challenges regarding their systemic administration and stability in the blood vascular system. In this regard, nanoparticles are demonstrating unique properties that may make this tool applicable as an advanced delivery vehicle. In this study, we have discussed various challenges for the use of bare siRNAs in the human body. We have also discussed the methods that may be used to fabricate the nanoparticles in order to deliver siRNAs. Moreover, we have included several nanoparticle conjugates with their advantages and disadvantages while using them as a delivery vehicle.

Keywords: Blood-brain barrier, Carbon-based nanoconjugate, Carbon nanotube, Cyclodextrin, Dendrimer, Endocytosis, Gold nanoparticle, Gene silencing, Graphene, Hydrogel nanoparticle, Immune response, Intravenous administration, Lipid-based nanoconjugate, Magnetic nanoparticle, Metal oxide nanoparticles, Polymer, Quantum dot nanoparticle, Silica-based nanoparticles, Systemic administration, Theranostic.

INTRODUCTION

Gene silencing is recognized as a prominent feature of eukaryotic organisms. siRNAs are one of the tools that silence the expression of the gene. siRNAs produce RNA-induced silencing complex (RISC) that degrades the double-stranded RNAs. This is the way how mRNAs are degraded and protein synthesis does not occur. siRNAs in their regular laboratory uses make them an important tool for determining the function of genes and their application in therapeutics (Fig. **1**). In this study, we intended to identify the challenges and hurdles of using bare siRNAs in the human body. Moreover, to determine the use of siRNA-nanoparticle conjugates with their advantages and disadvantages when used in the human body.

Rituparna Acharya

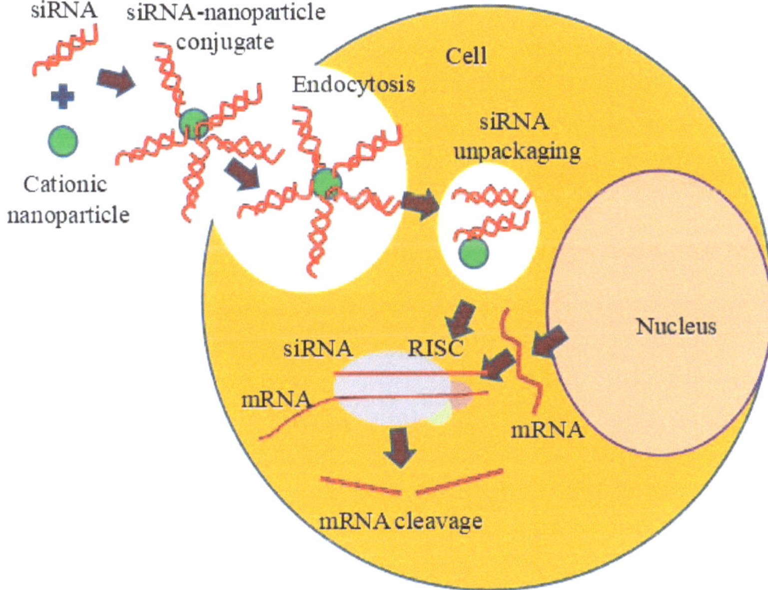

Fig. (1). Mechanism of action of siRNA-nanoparticle conjugate.

siRNAs as Potential Therapeutics

Due to the rise of siRNA application, many difficult and incurable diseases have attained the possibility to cure. Especially diseases such as cancer, which develops due to the overexpression of certain genes [1 - 3]. With the help of siRNA therapy, these disease conditions can be approached and these genes can be targeted as a therapeutic intervention. siRNAs may target any mRNA independent of their location and organ or structure of the translated protein. Therefore, siRNA therapy is increasingly becoming a promising agent for meeting the challenges and becoming a new generation bio-drug.

Significant progress has been made on siRNA silencing property for therapeutic applications. Currently, many siRNA based drugs are under clinical trial.

CHALLENGES IN DELIVERY OF SIRNA

siRNA therapy is built on the concept of "loss of function". siRNAs are actually involved in the silencing of the mRNA that prevents the expression of protein from that specific mRNA. As siRNAs are not incorporated in the genome, they do not produce any permanent modification of the DNA within the cell. So, the siRNA therapy can be stopped at any point of time [4] but it has drawbacks of "off-target" effect when they are not efficiently targeted to the tissue/cell/organ.

siRNA delivery has several challenges such as enzymatic degradation in the blood when administered through intravenous injection, rapid renal clearance, phagocytosis by macrophage and other cells in the blood. Other challenges after reaching the target site are the challenge of overcoming vascular barriers such as blood-brain barrier, uptake of siRNA by target cells, release in the cytoplasm from endosome and release of the payload.

Administrative Barrier

Most of the disease target sites are not available for oral route. Moreover, the oral route has many drawbacks such as special precautions should be taken to maintain intestinal stability and for better permeability through the intestinal epithelium [5]. On the other hand, subcutaneous injection is another route of administration that overcomes the hurdles of permeability through intestinal epithelium but subcutaneous injection also has some disadvantages such as the siRNA in the blood may come across the phagocytic cells of the immune system and siRNA may undergo phagocytosis by them. However, the most commonly applied injections for siRNAs are intravenous injections.

Vascular Barrier

To reach the target site crossing the vascular endothelium is a crucial step. Further, the renal clearance through glomerular filtration is another challenge for siRNAs [6]. Moreover, the protection of siRNAs from phagocytic cells is another hurdle for the therapeutic use of these macromolecules [7].

Cellular Barriers

The next important challenge of cellular uptake of siRNAs is that cell membranes are composed of negatively charged protein and lipid layers. As siRNAs are also negatively charged so, the repulsion of the charges takes place on the surface of the cell membrane. This prevents siRNAs to internalize within the cell. The next important challenge is the successful endosomal escape of the siRNA in the cytoplasm [8].

Immune Response and Safety

The most important challenge of this category is that siRNAs should not produce any immunogenic response in the body and should refrain from any undesirable side effect. There should be no off-target gene silencing in the normal cells of the body [9, 10]. Moreover, the innate immune system of our body should not recognize the siRNA as a foreign particle before reaching it to the target site [11, 12].

OVERCOMING THE MAJOR BARRIERS FOR siRNA DELIVERY

The DNA delivery system as described in the previous section is different from siRNA delivery vehicles in many respects [13]. Although the anionic nature of the DNA and RNAs are similar but the plasmid DNA with several thousands of base pairs are much larger in size than siRNAs that are only 21-23 base pair long. Over the past several years many strategies are designed for optimum delivery of siRNA having these differences in mind.

Intravenous Administration

Intravenous administration overcomes the barrier of intestinal instability due to the presence of acidic environment in the stomach and alkaline environment in the small intestine. Moreover, this type of administration doesn't need any intestinal absorption as it directly meets to the blood.

Optimization of the Size of the siRNA Nanocarrier

To reach the target site the major hurdles is to be permeable to the vascular endothelium layer of the blood vessels. In respect to this challenge the size of the nanocarriers are controlled up to 100nm so that they can easily pass the blood endothelial barrier and come into contact with the cells.

Moreover, in the kidney glomerular filtration takes place that can again clear the siRNA nanoconjugate from the blood. The pore size of the glomerular filtration barrier is 8nm. So, to address this problem the size of the nanoconjugate should be approximately 20nm [14, 15].

Further, large sized nanocarriers are susceptible to phagocytosis. Excessive net charge leads to aggregation so minimum net charge is required to maintain the stability in the blood. Lipophilicity increases uptake of the siRNA nanoparticle conjugate by the cells [16].

Endocytosis of siRNA-nanoparticle Conjugate

For internalization of the nanoconjugate endocytosis method is adopted that may be receptor mediated endocytosis which is driven by several common ligands such as folate [17], transferrin [18] and aptamer [19].

Further, the endosomal escape of the nanocarrier can be enhanced by cationic polymer that increases the endosomolysis of the membrane of endosomes [20]. However, the mechanism of endosomal delivery is poorly understood, so, more research in this area will reveal in avenues of the delivery of siRNAs.

Overcoming the Immune Response

This challenge of the siRNAs identified as a foreign particle by the immune system can be addressed by restricting the length of siRNAs to 21-23 nucleotides long [11] or by modifying the siRNA at 2′-O-methylation.

NANOPARTICLE IN SIRNA THERAPY

Development of nanoparticles using nanotechnology is from last few years are for the diagnostic and therapeutic applications. In comparison with the traditional medicines nanoparticle can overcome many hurdles of application that are discussed in the previous section. The most remarkable property of the nanoparticles is to protect its payload from enzymatic degradation in the blood and hiding them from phagocytes. Moreover, they make the siRNA highly permeable through the blood vascular endothelium and through cell membrane. Current research area is highly focused on the optimization of the size, shape, surface chemistry, concentration and composition of the nanoparticles [21].

Further, more research is currently going on nanoparticles that can have a stable association with the siRNAs. Limited success has been achieved and more challenges are on the stability and toxicity *in vivo*. Wide variety of nanoparticles has advantages as well as drawbacks when associated with siRNA in their physiochemical properties and compositions. Here in this study we are intended to discuss the advantages and disadvantages of the nanoparticles in conjugation with siRNA and their current state of development.

siRNA-silica Based Nanoconjugate

Silica and silicon based nanoparticles are emerging as a novel drug delivery vehicle for their controllability on nanopore formulation and surface modification. Various spherical mesoporous silica nanoparticles are also used for the delivery of siRNAs to the target organ. They have several advantages are follows [22 - 27]:

- Mesoporous silica nanoparticles have large surface area that increases the surface to volume ratio.
- In this nanoparticle the siRNAs are stable.
- These conjugates are highly biocompatible and biodegradable as well.
- The porosity of the mesoporous silica nanoparticles is highly controllable and that allows the multifunctional and sequential delivery of the siRNAs.
- Mesoporous silica nanoparticles have high surface reactivity and easy functionalization by siRNAs.

The only disadvantage of this nanoconjugate is as follows [28]:

- This nanoconjugate demonstrates toxicity while *in vivo* experiments.

siRNA-metal and Metal Oxide Nanoconjugates

Different types of nanoparticles are tested so far for siRNA delivery purposes. Among them, magnetic nanoparticles have received increased attention in this field. By the help of magnetic field transfection is performed that increases the cellular transport process [29]. The main advantages of magnetic nanoparticles in conjugation with siRNAs are as follows [30 - 32]:

- They have large surface area.
- As they are smaller in size they have improved tissue permeability and remains in circulation for longer period of time.
- Remote controlled and fast delivery of siRNA through magnetic field.
- These types of nanoconjugates do not agglomerate.
- They have wide variety of applications such as targeting, diagnosis and therapy.

The drawbacks of magnetic nanoconjugates are as follows [33]:

- This type of nanoconjugate have low colloidal stability.
- They are sometimes proved to be cytotoxic and have limited biocompatibility.
- Moreover, they are non-biodegradable.

Another metallic nanoparticlc is gold nanoparticle that is highly biocompatible and easy to synthesis and can be easily conjugated with variety of siRNAs [34].

The main advantages are as follows [35]:

- Gold nanoparticles have high surface to volume ratio.
- These nanoconjugates are easy to synthesis, easy to modify their surface properties and easy to conjugate with siRNAs.
- They are highly biocompatible.
- The siRNA-gold nanoconjugates are stable in their structure.

The disadvantages of siRNA-gold nanoconjugates are as follows:

- Gold nanoparticles are highly expensive for mass production.
- They are instable when used in *in vivo* applications.
- Gold nanoconjugates are non-biodegradable.

siRNA-carbon Based Nanoconjugates

Carbon nanotube and graphine nanosheets as allotropic nanostructures have created enormous attention in gene delivery and siRNA therapeutic applications. Their nanoscale needle structure is efficiently taken up by the cells [36 - 38]. The main advantages of carbon nanotubes are [39, 40]:

- They have large surface areas to attach with wide variety of ligands.
- It has a high loading capacity of siRNAs and other payloads and has high functionalizing capacity.
- Carbon nanotubes have high permeability to biological systems such as blood brain barriers *etc.*
- They have high mechanical strength and thermal and electrical conductivity.
- They can easily encapsulate and store the delivery molecule within them.

The main drawbacks are [41]:

- Carbon nanotubes are difficult in mass production and handling.
- They may be toxic in certain cells.
- Carbon nanotubes are non-biodegradable in their property.

The newly discovered carbon nanosheet 2-dimensional structure is graphene [42 - 44]. It is a novel nanocarrier of siRNAs. The advantages of graphene are as follows [45, 46]:

- Graphene nanosheets have large surface area.
- They have facile synthesis method.
- They are stable as colloidal structures.
- They can be easily functionalized at their surface.
- Lastly they have a good mechanical and electrical property.

The disadvantages of graphene nanosheets are as follows [47]:

- Graphene nanosheets are highly costly.

- The mass production of graphene is difficult.
- There are safety concerns of grapheme while their application.
- They are highly non-biodegradable.

siRNA-dendrimer Nanoconjugates

Dendrimers are symmetrical branch molecules with a central core. They have controllable size and shape [48, 49] that can deliver a wide variety of molecules including DNA and siRNAs. The advantages of these dendrimers are as follows:

- The size and shape of dendrimers may be precisely controllable.
- They are highly water soluble.
- Dendrimers are biocompatible and non-toxic.
- When administered in the human body they produce negligible immune responses.
- siRNA-Dendrimers have negligible nuclease activity when administered in the blood.
- siRNA and dendrimers have electrostatic interaction within them.

The drawbacks of siRNA-dendrimers are as follows [50]:

- This nanoconjugate has demonstrated non-specific cytotoxicity.
- The dendrimer have limited release of siRNAs within the cell.
- The conjugate undergo rapid clearance from the blood.

siRNA-polymer Nanoconjugate

Unit by unit construction makes the polymers that may be fabricated so that they can become an efficient transfection agent of siRNAs and may release the payload when needed. Extensively the polymers are been reviewed [13, 51, 52] and they have a wide variety of polymers including synthetic and natural in their composition. The polymers have several advantages such as [53, 54]:

- They are easy and cheap to produce in bulk.
- Optimum fabrication methods may be used for fine tuning of the structure and properties of the particles.
- They have simple procedure for loading siRNAs with electrostatic interaction.
- They can be formulated in wide range of molecular weights.
- Polymers that are natural in their composition are usually biocompatible, non-toxic and biodegradable.

The disadvantages of polymers in conjugation with siRNAs are as follows [55]:

- The siRNA-polymer nanoconjugates have a limited stability in the blood.
- The polymers that are synthetic in their composition usually cause cellular apoptosis and necrosis.

siRNA-Cyclodextrin Nanoconjugate

Cyclic polysaccharides are the building blocks of the cyclodextrin nanoparticles. Due to their high biocompatibility they are used for wide range of applications in medicine [56, 57]. The main advantages are as follows [58]:

- Cyclodextrin have very low toxicity.
- They can easily intercalate the biological macromolecules within their structure.
- siRNA-cyclodextrin usually don't produce any immune response in the body when administered.
- The nanoparticle easily protects its payload, so, siRNA do not get degraded in the blood when they are intercalated within the cyclodextrin nanoparticle.

The drawbacks of this nanoconjugate are as follows:

- The mass production of siRNA-cyclodextrin nanoconjugate is highly expensive.
- There are concerns regarding their safety during production.
- This nanoconjugate is not easily soluble.

siRNA-lipid Based Nanoconjugates

The most advanced and highly studied nanoparticle is liposomal nanoparticles. They are widely used in clinical application [59 - 62] and are in clinical trials and are approved by FDA [63 - 65]. Followings are the advantages of siRNA-lipid based nanoconjugates when they are used in clinical applications [66]:

- These nanoconjugates are highly biocompatible and non-toxic to human body.
- Due to their structural properties they are rapidly taken up by the cells and cellular uptake is easy.
- They may be easily fabricated while synthesis and formulation.
- This nanoconjugate may be targeted to the site of action very easily and can release the payload in a controlled release pattern.
- Liposomal nanoparticles may be conjugated with siRNAs, ligands, probes and fluorophores very easily.

The drawbacks of the use of siRNA-liposomal nanoconjugates are as follows:

- These nanoconjugates have a very high production cost.
- Sometimes this nanoconjugate may demonstrate leakage of the payload and instability within the body.
- The conjugates have low solubility.
- Lastly, they are rapidly cleared from the blood by glomerular filtration.

siRNA-hydrogel Nanoconjugate

Hydrogels are 3-dimensional polymeric material that may retain a large amount of water and biological fluid material. They may be macroscopic, microscopic and nanogels [67, 68]. Currently, nanogel materials are of intense investigation for biomedical application. The main advantages of the nanoconjugates are [69, 70]:

- They have tenable synthesis and physiochemical properties.
- Their surface may be functionalized selectively.
- Due to their highly porous structure, they have a high loading capacity of the payload.
- The release of the payload is highly controlled and has sustained release capacity to the target tissue.
- These nanoconjugates are highly biocompatible and biodegradable.

The disadvantages of the use of this nanoconjugate are as follows:

- The mass production of these nanoconjugates is highly expensive.
- The siRNA-hydrogel nanoconjugate is not stable within the human body.

siRNA-quantum Dot Nanoconjugate

Quantum dot is considered to be an efficient theranostic tool due to its size, structure and photo chemical stability. It is considered as a new generation nanoparticle that has diagnostic applications with fluorescence imaging [71 - 74] and therapeutic property [71, 75 - 78]. The main advantages are as follows:

- They can be fabricated depending upon their size and structure for diagnostic purposes.
- These nanoconjugates have high molar extinction coefficient.

- They have high photo and chemical stability while diagnosis and therapeutic applications.
- siRNA-quantum dot nanoconjugates have synergistic and diagnostic and therapeutic applications.

The drawbacks are as follows [79]:

- Quantum dot nanoparticles have toxicity in the body when applied.
- They degrade easily within the system.
- They have a potential aggregation tendency.
- Lastly, they are removed from the body easily.

CONCLUSION

The dynamic property of nanoparticles influences the association and dissociation curve of cells in the body fluid. Nanoparticles after establishment of contact with the biological environment cover the cells that are known as "halo". The dynamic response of nanoparticles is determined by the concentration of protein in the biological fluid and construction of this "halo". The unhealthy fluids bring remarkable changes in the dynamic nature of the nanoparticles. The mechanical properties of the unhealthy fluid produce a reasonable response in the nanoparticle [80].

siRNA-nanoparticle conjugates are considered to be the most potent therapeutic in the medicinal application. However, to make them optimum in their applications, more research in this field is required. Many challenges and barriers should be addressed before it becomes an optimum drug molecule in today's world. Systemic delivery of siRNAs is the major challenge today. In this respect, nanoparticle-mediated delivery is emerging as a potent technology. A wide variety of nanoparticles has their advantages and drawbacks while administering in the human body due to their different physiochemical properties. They have a range of effectiveness when they are used in conjugation with siRNAs.

Silica nanoparticles may deliver large payloads due to their controllable porosity. Magnetic nanoparticles have unique properties that make them a theranostic agent. Carbon nanostructures due to their shape and size may penetrate the cell walls easily. As liposomes are made of lipid particles, they are highly biocompatible. Moreover, hydrogels have a highly porous structure that makes them an ideal controlled delivery and makes them carry high molecular weight payloads. Unit by unit construction of polymers makes them an efficient transfection and release nanoparticle.

These unique properties of the nanoparticles make them efficient in siRNA delivery to the cells and target organs. However, success will be achieved only after overcoming the barriers associated with other stages of delivery. Further, research is necessary to develop an optimum nanoparticle with unique properties that may deliver siRNA in an optimum way. The development of novel nanoparticles with ideal nanostructures can subsequently make the siRNA delivery a true potential for therapy.

REFERENCES

[1] Chin K, DeVries S, Fridlyand J, Spellman PT, Roydasgupta R, Kuo W-L, *et al.* Genomic and transcriptional aberrations linked to breast cancer pathophysiologies. Cancer Cell 2006; 10(6): 529-41. [http://dx.doi.org/10.1016/j.ccr.2006.10.009]

[2] Xu J, Chen Y, Olopade OI. MYC and breast cancer. Genes Cancer 2010; 1(6): 629-40. [http://dx.doi.org/10.1177/1947601910378691] [PMID: 21779462]

[3] Onel K, Cordon-Cardo C. MDM2 and prognosis. Mol Cancer Res 2004; 2(1): 1-8. [PMID: 14757840]

[4] Resnier P, Montier T, Mathieu V, Benoit JP, Passirani C. A review of the current status of siRNA nanomedicines in the treatment of cancer. Biomaterials 2013; 34(27): 6429-43. [http://dx.doi.org/10.1016/j.biomaterials.2013.04.060] [PMID: 23727262]

[5] Haussecker D. Current issues of RNAi therapeutics delivery and development. J Cont Rel 2014; 195: 49-54. [http://dx.doi.org/10.1016/j.jconrel.2014.07.056] [PMID: 25111131]

[6] Jarad G, Miner JH. Update on the glomerular filtration barrier. Curr Opin Nephrol Hypertens 2009; 18(3): 226-32. [http://dx.doi.org/10.1097/MNH.0b013e3283296044] [PMID: 19374010]

[7] Moghimi SM, Hunter AC, Murray JC. Long-circulating and target-specific nanoparticles: theory to practice. Pharmacol Rev 2001; 53(2): 283-318. [PMID: 11356986]

[8] Meade BR, Dowdy SF. Exogenous siRNA delivery using peptide transduction domains/cell penetrating peptides. Adv Drug Deliv Rev 2007; 59(2-3): 134-40. [http://dx.doi.org/10.1016/j.addr.2007.03.004] [PMID: 17451840]

[9] Jackson AL, Burchard J, Schelter J, *et al.* Widespread siRNA "off-target" transcript silencing mediated by seed region sequence complementarity. RNA 2006; 12(7): 1179-87. [http://dx.doi.org/10.1261/rna.25706] [PMID: 16682560]

[10] Qiu S, Adema CM, Lane T. A computational study of off-target effects of RNA interference. Nucleic Acids Res 2005; 33(6): 1834-47. [http://dx.doi.org/10.1093/nar/gki324] [PMID: 15800213]

[11] Hornung V, Guenthner-Biller M, Bourquin C, *et al.* Sequence-specific potent induction of IFN-alpha by short interfering RNA in plasmacytoid dendritic cells through TLR7. Nat Med 2005; 11(3): 263-70. [http://dx.doi.org/10.1038/nm1191] [PMID: 15723075]

[12] Judge AD, Sood V, Shaw JR, Fang D, McClintock K, MacLachlan I. Sequence-dependent stimulation of the mammalian innate immune response by synthetic siRNA. Nat Biotechnol 2005; 23(4): 457-62. [http://dx.doi.org/10.1038/nbt1081] [PMID: 15778705]

[13] Gary DJ, Puri N, Won YY. Polymer-based siRNA delivery: perspectives on the fundamental and phenomenological distinctions from polymer-based DNA delivery. J Cont Rel Soc 2007; 121(1-2): 64-73.

[http://dx.doi.org/10.1016/j.jconrel.2007.05.021] [PMID: 17588702]

[14] Wartiovaara J, Ofverstedt LG, Khoshnoodi J, *et al.* Nephrin strands contribute to a porous slit diaphragm scaffold as revealed by electron tomography. J Clin Invest 2004; 114(10): 1475-83. [http://dx.doi.org/10.1172/JCI22562] [PMID: 15545998]

[15] Huang Y, Hong J, Zheng S, Ding Y, Guo S, Zhang H, *et al.* Elimination pathways of systemically delivered siRNA. Molecular Therapy: J Amer Soc Gene Therapy 2011 ; 19(2): 381-5. [http://dx.doi.org/10.1038/mt.2010.266] [PMID: 21119623]

[16] Huang K, Ma H, Liu J, Huo S, Kumar A, Wei T, *et al.* Size-dependent localization and penetration of ultrasmall gold nanoparticles in cancer cells, multicellular spheroids, and tumors *in vivo*. ACS Nano 2012; 6(5): 4483-93.

[17] Rozema DB, Lewis DL, Wakefield DH, Wong SC, Klein JJ, Roesch PL, *et al.* Dynamic polyconjugates for targeted *in vivo* delivery of siRNA to hepatocytes. Proc Natl Acad Sci USA. 104(32): 12982-7. [http://dx.doi.org/10.1073/pnas.0703778104]

[18] Konishi M, Kawamoto K, Izumikawa M, Kuriyama H, Yamashita T. Gene transfer into guinea pig cochlea using adeno-associated virus vectors. J Gene Med 2008; 10(6): 610-8. [http://dx.doi.org/10.1002/jgm.1189] [PMID: 18338819]

[19] Chu TC, Twu KY, Ellington AD, Levy M. Aptamer mediated siRNA delivery. Nucleic Acids Res 2006; 34(10): e73. [http://dx.doi.org/10.1093/nar/gkl388] [PMID: 16740739]

[20] Appelqvist H, Wäster P, Kågedal K, Öllinger K. The lysosome: from waste bag to potential therapeutic target. J Mol Cell Biol 2013; 5(4): 214-26. [http://dx.doi.org/10.1093/jmcb/mjt022] [PMID: 23918283]

[21] Jiang W, Kim BY, Rutka JT, Chan WC. Nanoparticle-mediated cellular response is size-dependent. Nat Nanotechnol 2008; 3(3): 145-50. [http://dx.doi.org/10.1038/nnano.2008.30] [PMID: 18654486]

[22] Tasciotti E, Liu X, Bhavane R, Plant K, Leonard A, Price B, *et al.* Mesoporous silicon particles as a multistage delivery system for imaging and therapeutic applications. Nature Nanotechnology 2008; 3: 151-7. [http://dx.doi.org/10.1038/nnano.2008.34]

[23] Serda RE, Godin B, Blanco E, Chiappini C, Ferrari M. Multi-stage delivery nano-particle systems for therapeutic applications. Biochim Biophys Acta 2011; 1810(3): 317-29. [http://dx.doi.org/10.1016/j.bbagen.2010.05.004] [PMID: 20493927]

[24] Meng H, Xue M, Xia T, *et al.* Use of size and a copolymer design feature to improve the biodistribution and the enhanced permeability and retention effect of doxorubicin-loaded mesoporous silica nanoparticles in a murine xenograft tumor model. ACS Nano 2011; 5(5): 4131-44. [http://dx.doi.org/10.1021/nn200809t] [PMID: 21524062]

[25] Cauda V, Schlossbauer A, Bein T. Bio-degradation study of colloidal mesoporous silica nanoparticles: Effect of surface functionalization with organo-silanes and poly(ethylene glycol). Microporous and Mesoporous Materials 2010; 132(1): 60-71.

[26] Souris JS, Lee CH, Cheng SH, *et al.* Surface charge-mediated rapid hepatobiliary excretion of mesoporous silica nanoparticles. Biomaterials 2010; 31(21): 5564-74. [http://dx.doi.org/10.1016/j.biomaterials.2010.03.048] [PMID: 20417962]

[27] Rosenholm JM, Mamaeva V, Sahlgren C, Lindén M. Nanoparticles in targeted cancer therapy: mesoporous silica nanoparticles entering preclinical development stage. Nanomedicine (Lond) 2012; 7(1): 111-20. [http://dx.doi.org/10.2217/nnm.11.166] [PMID: 22191780]

[28] Zhang H, Dunphy DR, Jiang X, *et al.* Processing pathway dependence of amorphous silica

nanoparticle toxicity: colloidal *vs* pyrolytic. J Am Chem Soc 2012; 134(38): 15790-804. [http://dx.doi.org/10.1021/ja304907c] [PMID: 22924492]

[29] Park JW, Bae KH, Kim C, Park TG. Clustered magnetite nanocrystals cross-linked with PEI for efficient siRNA delivery. Biomacromolecules 2011; 12(2): 457-65. [http://dx.doi.org/10.1021/bm101244j] [PMID: 21190334]

[30] Boussif O, Lezoualc'h F, Zanta MA, Mergny MD, Scherman D, Demeneix B, *et al.* A versatile vector for gene and oligonucleotide transfer into cells in culture and *in vivo*: polyethylenimine. Proc Natl Acad Sci USA. 92(16): 7297-301. [http://dx.doi.org/10.1073/pnas.92.16.7297]

[31] Park JW, Mok H, Park TG. Epidermal growth factor (EGF) receptor targeted delivery of PEGylated adenovirus. Biochem Biophys Res Commun 2008; 366(3): 769-74. [http://dx.doi.org/10.1016/j.bbrc.2007.12.045] [PMID: 18083120]

[32] Mok H, Park TG. Self-crosslinked and reducible fusogenic peptides for intracellular delivery of siRNA. Biopolymers 2008; 89(10): 881-8. [http://dx.doi.org/10.1002/bip.21032] [PMID: 18521895]

[33] Schrand AM, Rahman MF, Hussain SM, Schlager JJ, Smith DA, Syed AF. Metal-based nanoparticles and their toxicity assessment. Wiley Interdiscip Rev Nanomed Nanobiotechnol 2010; 2(5): 544-68. [http://dx.doi.org/10.1002/wnan.103] [PMID: 20681021]

[34] Boisselier E, Astruc D. Gold nanoparticles in nanomedicine: preparations, imaging, diagnostics, therapies and toxicity. Chem Soc Rev 2009; 38(6): 1759-82. [http://dx.doi.org/10.1039/b806051g] [PMID: 19587967]

[35] Khlebtsov N, Dykman L. Biodistribution and toxicity of engineered gold nanoparticles: a review of *in vitro* and *in vivo* studies. Chem Soc Rev 2011; 40(3): 1647-71. [http://dx.doi.org/10.1039/C0CS00018C] [PMID: 21082078]

[36] Ji Z, Lin G, Lu Q, *et al.* Targeted therapy of SMMC-7721 liver cancer in vitro and in vivo with carbon nanotubes based drug delivery system. J Colloid Interface Sci 2012; 365(1): 143-9. [http://dx.doi.org/10.1016/j.jcis.2011.09.013] [PMID: 21974923]

[37] Pantarotto D, Briand JP, Prato M, Bianco A. Translocation of bioactive peptides across cell membranes by carbon nanotubes. Chem Commun 2004; 16-7. [PMID: 14737310]

[38] Pantarotto D, Singh R, McCarthy D, *et al.* Functionalized carbon nanotubes for plasmid DNA gene delivery. Angew Chem Int Ed Engl 2004; 43(39): 5242-6. [http://dx.doi.org/10.1002/anie.200460437] [PMID: 15455428]

[39] Liu Z, Tabakman SM, Chen Z, Dai H. Preparation of carbon nanotube bioconjugates for biomedical applications. Nat Protoc 2009; 4(9): 1372-82. [http://dx.doi.org/10.1038/nprot.2009.146] [PMID: 19730421]

[40] Dervishi E, Li Z, Xu Y, Saini V, Biris AR, Lupu D, *et al.* Carbon nanotubes: synthesis, properties, and applications. Part Sci Technol 2009; 27(2): 107-25.

[41] Beguin F, Ehrburger P. Special issue on carbon nanotubes. Carbon 2002; 40: 1619.

[42] Novoselov KS, Geim AK, Morozov SV, *et al.* Electric field effect in atomically thin carbon films. Science 2004; 306(5696): 666-9. [http://dx.doi.org/10.1126/science.1102896] [PMID: 15499015]

[43] Geim AK, Novoselov KS. The rise of graphene. Nat Mater 2007; 6(3): 183-91. [http://dx.doi.org/10.1038/nmat1849] [PMID: 17330084]

[44] Li X, Wang X, Zhang L, Lee S, Dai H. Chemically derived, ultrasmooth graphene nanoribbon semiconductors. Science 2008; 319(5867): 1229-32.

[http://dx.doi.org/10.1126/science.1150878] [PMID: 18218865]

[45] Li D, Müller M, Gilje S, Kaner R, Wallace G. Processable aqueous dispersion of graphene nanosheets. Nat. Nanotechnol 2008; 3: 101-5.
[http://dx.doi.org/10.1038/nnano.2007.451]

[46] Feng L, Zhang S, Liu Z. Graphene based gene transfection. Nanoscale 2011; 3(3): 1252-7.
[http://dx.doi.org/10.1039/c0nr00680g] [PMID: 21270989]

[47] Seabra AB, Paula AJ, de Lima R, Alves OL, Durán N. Nanotoxicity of graphene and graphene oxide. Chem Res Toxicol 2014; 27(2): 159-68.
[http://dx.doi.org/10.1021/tx400385x] [PMID: 24422439]

[48] Biswas S, Torchilin VP. Dendrimers for siRNA delivery. Pharmaceuticals (Basel) 2013; 6(2): 161-83.
[http://dx.doi.org/10.3390/ph6020161] [PMID: 24275946]

[49] Wu J, Huang W, He Z. Dendrimers as carriers for siRNA delivery and gene silencing: a review. Sci World J 2013; 630654.
[http://dx.doi.org/10.1155/2013/630654] [PMID: 24288498]

[50] Duncan R, Izzo L. Dendrimer biocompatibility and toxicity. Adv Drug Deliv Rev 2005; 57(15): 2215-37.
[http://dx.doi.org/10.1016/j.addr.2005.09.019] [PMID: 16297497]

[51] Liu XQ, Sun CY, Yang XZ, Wang J. Polymeric-micelle-based nanomedicine for siRNA delivery. Part Part Syst Charact 2013; 30(3): 211-28.
[http://dx.doi.org/10.1039/9781849737388-00158]

[52] Oh Y-K, Park TG. siRNA delivery systems for cancer treatment. Adv. Drug Deliv. Rev 2009; 61(10): 850-62.

[53] Lee SJ, Huh MS, Lee SY, *et al.* Tumor-homing poly-siRNA/glycol chitosan self-cross-linked nanoparticles for systemic siRNA delivery in cancer treatment. Angew Chem Int Ed Engl 2012; 51(29): 7203-7.
[http://dx.doi.org/10.1002/anie.201201390] [PMID: 22696263]

[54] Yang J, Li S, Guo F, Zhang W, Wang Y, Pan Y. Induction of apoptosis by chitosan/HPV16 E7 siRNA complexes in cervical cancer cells. Mol Med Rep 2013; 7(3): 998-1002.
[http://dx.doi.org/10.3892/mmr.2012.1246] [PMID: 23258711]

[55] Lee SY, Huh MS, Lee S, Lee SJ, Chung H, Park JH, *et al.* Stability and cellular uptake of polymerized siRNA (poly-siRNA)/polyethylenimine (PEI) complexes for efficient gene silencing. J. Cont Rel Soc 2010; 141(3): 339-46.
[PMID: 19836427]

[56] Kurkov SV, Loftsson T. Cyclodextrins. Int J Pharm 2013; 453(1): 167-80.
[http://dx.doi.org/10.1016/j.ijpharm.2012.06.055] [PMID: 22771733]

[57] Jansook P, Kurkov SV, Loftsson T. Cyclodextrins as solubilizers: formation of complex aggregates. J Pharm Sci 2010; 99(2): 719-29.
[http://dx.doi.org/10.1002/jps.21861] [PMID: 19670293]

[58] Tiwari G, Tiwari R, Rai AK. Cyclodextrins in delivery systems: Applications. J Pharm Bioallied Sci 2010; 2(2): 72-9.
[http://dx.doi.org/10.4103/0975-7406.67003] [PMID: 21814436]

[59] Hatakeyama H, Akita H, Ito E, *et al.* Systemic delivery of siRNA to tumors using a lipid nanoparticle containing a tumor-specific cleavable PEG-lipid. Biomaterials 2011; 32(18): 4306-16.
[http://dx.doi.org/10.1016/j.biomaterials.2011.02.045] [PMID: 21429576]

[60] Schroeder A, Levins CG, Cortez C, Langer R, Anderson DG. Lipid-based nanotherapeutics for siRNA delivery. J Intern Med 2010; 267(1): 9-21.
[http://dx.doi.org/10.1111/j.1365-2796.2009.02189.x] [PMID: 20059641]

[61] Tseng Y-C, Mozumdar S, Huang L. Lipid-based systemic delivery of siRNA. Adv Drug Deliv Rev 2009; 61(9): 721-31.
[PMID: 19328215] [http://dx.doi.org/10.1016/j.addr.2009.03.003]

[62] Allen TM, Cullis PR. Drug delivery systems: entering the mainstream. Science 2004; 303(5665): 1818-22.
[http://dx.doi.org/10.1126/science.1095833] [PMID: 15031496]

[63] Noble CO, Guo Z, Hayes MF, Marks JD, Park JW, Benz CC, *et al.* Characterization of highly stable liposomal and immunoliposomal formulations of vincristine and vinblastine. Cancer Chemother Pharmacol 2009; 64(4): 741-51.
[http://dx.doi.org/10.1007/s00280-008-0923-3] [PMID: 19184019]

[64] Drummond D, Noble C, Guo Z, Hayes M, Connolly-Ingram C, Gabriel B, *et al.* Development of a highly stable and targetable nanoliposomal formulation of topotecan. J Control Rel: Official J Control Rel Soc 2009; 141: 13-21.

[65] Lin Q, Chen J, Zhang Z, Zheng G. Lipid-based nanoparticles in the systemic delivery of siRNA. Nanomedicine (Lond) 2014; 9(1): 105-20.
[http://dx.doi.org/10.2217/nnm.13.192] [PMID: 24354813]

[66] Lv H, Zhang S, Wang B, Cui S, Yan J. Toxicity of cationic lipids and cationic polymers in gene delivery. J Control Rel Soc 2006; 114(1): 100-9.
[http://dx.doi.org/10.1016/j.jconrel.2006.04.014] [PMID: 16831482]

[67] Peppas NA, Bures P, Leobandung W, Ichikawa H. Hydrogels in pharmaceutical formulations. Eur J Pharm Biopharm 2000; 50(1): 27-46.
[http://dx.doi.org/10.1016/S0939-6411(00)00090-4] [PMID: 10840191]

[68] Raemdonck K, Thienen T, Vandenbroucke R, Sanders N, Demeester J, De Smedt S. Dextran microgels for time-controlled delivery of siRNA. Adv Funct Mater 2008; 18(7): 993-1001.
[http://dx.doi.org/10.1002/adfm.200701039]

[69] Peppas N, Hilt J, Khademhosseini A, Langer R. Hydrogels in biology and medicine: from molecular principles to bionanotechnology. Advan Mater 2006; 18(11): 1345-60.

[70] Ramakrishnan S. Hydrogel-siRNA for cancer therapy. Cancer Biol Ther 2011; 11(9): 849-51.
[http://dx.doi.org/10.4161/cbt.11.9.15465] [PMID: 21436621]

[71] Derfus AM, Chen AA, Min DH, Ruoslahti E, Bhatia SN. Targeted quantum dot conjugates for siRNA delivery. Bioconjug Chem 2007; 18(5): 1391-6.
[http://dx.doi.org/10.1021/bc060367e] [PMID: 17630789]

[72] Alivisatos AP. Semiconductor clusters, nanocrystals, and quantum dots. Science 1996; 271(5251): 933-7.
[http://dx.doi.org/10.1126/science.271.5251.933]

[73] Clapp AR, Medintz IL, Mauro JM, Fisher BR, Bawendi MG, Mattoussi H. Fluorescence resonance energy transfer between quantum dot donors and dye-labeled protein acceptors. J Am Chem Soc 2004; 126(1): 301-10.
[http://dx.doi.org/10.1021/ja037088b] [PMID: 14709096]

[74] Gao X, Cui Y, Levenson RM, Chung LW, Nie S. *In vivo* cancer targeting and imaging with semiconductor quantum dots. Nat Biotechnol 2004; 22(8): 969-76.
[http://dx.doi.org/10.1038/nbt994] [PMID: 15258594]

[75] Qi L, Gao X. Quantum dot-amphipol nanocomplex for intracellular delivery and real-time imaging of siRNA. ACS Nano 2008; 2(7): 1403-10.
[http://dx.doi.org/10.1021/nn800280r] [PMID: 19206308]

[76] Yezhelyev MV, Qi L, O'Regan RM, Nie S, Gao X. Proton-sponge coated quantum dots for siRNA

delivery and intracellular imaging. J Am Chem Soc 2008; 130(28): 9006-12. [http://dx.doi.org/10.1021/ja800086u]

[77] Lee H, Kim IK, Park TG. Intracellular trafficking and unpacking of siRNA/quantum dot-PEI complexes modified with and without cell penetrating peptide: confocal and flow cytometric FRET analysis. Bioconjug Chem 2010; 21(2): 289-95. [http://dx.doi.org/10.1021/bc900342p] [PMID: 20078095]

[78] Probst CE, Zrazhevskiy P, Bagalkot V, Gao X. Quantum dots as a platform for nanoparticle drug delivery vehicle design. Adv Drug Deliv Rev 2013; 65(5): 703-18. [http://dx.doi.org/10.1016/j.addr.2012.09.036] [PMID: 23000745]

[79] Hardman R. A toxicologic review of quantum dots: toxicity depends on physicochemical and environmental factors. Environ Health Perspect 2006; 114(2): 165-72. [http://dx.doi.org/10.1289/ehp.8284] [PMID: 16451849]

[80] Morales-Bonilla S, Martines-Arano H, Torres-Torres D, Ochoa-Ortega G, Carrillo-Delgado C, Trejo-Valdez M, *et al.* Dynamic and plasmonic response exhibited by Au nanoparticles suspended in blood plasma and cerebrospinal fluids. J Mol Liquids 2019; 281: 1-8. [http://dx.doi.org/10.1016/j.molliq.2019.02.073]

CHAPTER 7

shRNA-Nanoparticle Conjugate as a Therapeutic Option

Abstract: The recent trend of gene therapy includes the RNAi therapeutic approach. RNAi therapy comprises the delivery of siRNA, shRNA and miRNA molecules to the cells for gene silencing. Among these types, shRNA is a more stable knockdown method. However, bare shRNA molecules are large and they can not penetrate the cell membrane due to their negative charge and also they are fragile and degradable by RNase enzymes in the body. To overcome these problems, nanoparticles play a vital role. They encapsulate the shRNA within their structure and protect them from degradation. The nanoparticles are sometimes positively charged so they readily penetrate the cell membrane and are internalized by the cell. These features of the nanoconjugate made them a potential therapeutic agent. In this study, we intended to discuss the wide variety of nanoconjugates and their applications in diseases.

Keywords: Chitosan nanoparticle, Cyclodextrin, Dendrimer nanoparticle, Gene therapy, Gold nanoparticle, Inorganic nanoparticle, Lipid nanoparticle, Luciferase, Magnetic nanoparticle, miRNA, Organic nanoparticle, Polymeric nanoparticle, PEG, PEI, PLGA, RNAi, shRNA, Silica nanoparticle, siRNA, Surviving.

INTRODUCTION

Gene therapy is the current treatment modality for the cure of several disease conditions without side effects. The traditional treatment methods have side effects and the synthetic molecules are synthesized outside the body that are chemical in nature and are not found in the body under normal circumstances. On the other hand, gene therapy uses the materials that are usually found in the body such as DNA and RNA molecules. So this gene therapy includes the RNAi therapy that is known as RNA interference therapy [1].

RNAi therapy includes treatment through different types of RNAs such as siRNA, shRNA and miRNA. In this study, we intended to focus on shRNAs and their application in conjugation with nanoparticles. shRNAs are nothing but 19-20 base pair long nucleotide sequence with 14-11 nucleotide long hairpin loop. After transfection, shRNA-plasmid is incorporated within the genome of the host cell

Rituparna Acharya

and start transcribing the pre-shRNA. This pre-shRNA is transported to the cytoplasm from the nucleus by Exportin 5. In the cytoplasm, they are processed by Dicer and loaded with RISC (RNA-induced silencing complex). Here the sense strand is degraded and the antisense strand directs RISC to the RNA molecules that have the complementary sequence with the shRNA and degrades them [2].

shRNAs have several advantages over other types of RNAi therapies. shRNAs are highly stable and their knockdown produces a stable cell line, on the other hand, siRNAs do not produce stable cell lines and need repeated transfection. Moreover, shRNAs are highly specific to their targets as they have complementary sequence specific to the mRNA molecules whereas miRNAs are not specific. The seed sequence of them may target multiple mRNA molecules from wide variety of genes [3].

Even though the shRNAs have several advantages, bare shRNAs have several drawbacks also. Bare shRNAs cannot enter the cell without lipofectamin or electroporation as they are of large size [4, 5]. Moreover, as these macromolecules are negatively charged, they cannot enter the cell through the negatively charged cell membranes. Further, when these shRNAs are injected into the bloodstream, they are readily degraded by the nuclease enzymes (Fig. **1**) [6]. In this respect, nanoparticles play a role, for example, they protect the shRNA molecules from enzymatic degradation in the blood, as some nanoparticles are positively charged they help these macromolecules to pass the cell membrane easily. In this study, we intended to discuss the wide variety of nanoparticles that have the capacity to deliver the shRNA to the target organ. The nanoparticles may be broadly classified into three types *i.e.,* inorganic nanoparticles, organic nanoparticles and polymeric nanoparticles.

shRNA-NANOPARTICLE CONJUGATES

Inorganic Nanoconjugates

Gold nanoparticles are a type of inorganic nanoparticles that help in the delivery of shRNA as gold nanoparticle-DNA oligonucleotide nanoconjugates. p53shRNA was delivered in HEK293 and Hela cell lines. Similarly, Mcl-1 shRNA was also delivered using gold nanoparticle to suppress the genetic expression [7]. Gold nanoparticle was also used to proliferate human periodontalligament stem cells (hPDLSC) using LRP5 shRNA [8].

Magnetic nanoparticles are another type of inorganic nanoparticles that have theranostic applications. In a study, good result was obtained on the co-delivery of Doxorubicin (DOX)and Special AT-rich binding protein (SATB1) shRNA using magnetic nanoparticle to combat gastric cancer [9]. Moreover, reverse multi drug resistance was demonstrated in human leukemia cell line on the delivery of MDR1 shRNA using Fe_3O_4 magnetic nanoparticle [10]. In lung cancer, tumor growth was significantly reduced by IGF-1RshRNA *in vivo* [11]. Bacterial magnetosomes were used to co-deliver doxorubicin and pHSP70-Plk1-shRNA that was found to be more effective in osteosarcoma [12]. Further, in Parkinson's disease, α-synucleinshRNA proved to be effective in repairing the neurodegeneration when magnetic nanoparticles are used with a coating of oleic acid molecules [13].

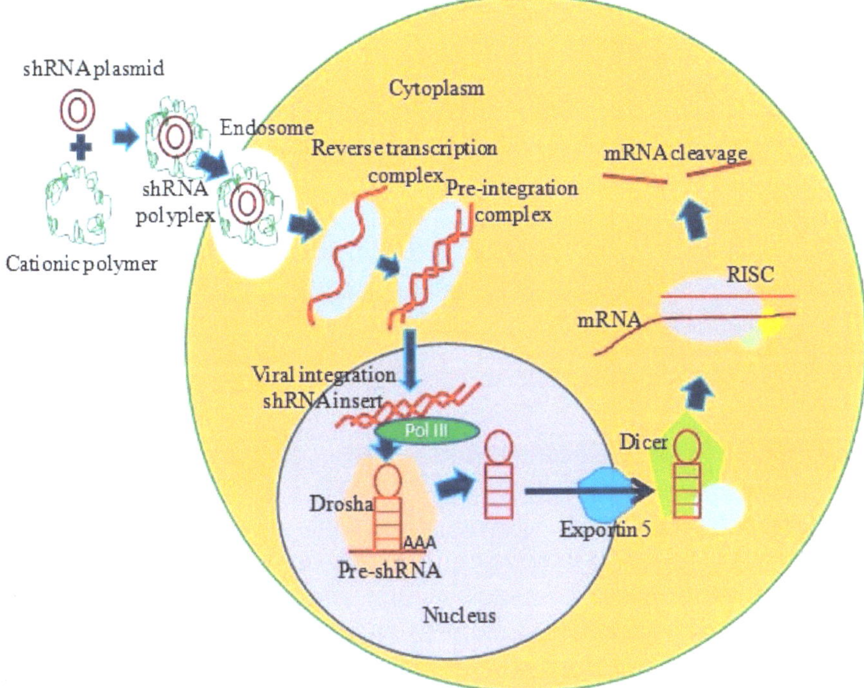

Fig. (1). Mechanism of action of shRNA plasmid-nanoparticle conjugate.

Silica nanoparticles are a variety of inorganic nanoparticles that helpin the inhibition of cancer growth and proliferation by using DOX and surviving shRNA [14]. Mesoporous silica nanoparticles are also a potent delivery vehicle for the co-delivery of DOX and pgpshRNA [15].

Organic Nanoconjugates

Among other types of organic nanoparticles, lipid nanoparticles are the most easily synthesizable, biocompatible and safe nanoparticle used in therapeutic applications. The solid lipid nanoparticles are potential delivery vehicle for the delivery of shRNAs. They are used for the inhibition of the viral protein of Hepatitis C virus by shRNA74 [16]. This nanoparticle is also used to inhibit 5-α reductase (p5α-Red) by shRNA-plasmid in human prostate cancer cell line [17]. *in vivo* HCV protein expression was also studied by using sshRNAs (short synthetic shRNAs) [18]. Inhibition of tumor cell proliferation, tumor cell apoptosis and reduction of the tumor weight was also documented by using shRNAs in conjugation with liposomal nanoparticle in ovarian cancer [19]. Another publication documented the use of PbishRNA EWS/FLI1 lipoplex (LPX) for the treatment of type1 Ewing's sarcoma demonstrated dose related safely and tumor response [20].

Polymeric Nanoconjugates

Chitosan nanoparticles are a type of polymeric nanoparticles that often help in theranostic applications. A novel nanoconjugate was developed using polyethyleneimine (PEI)-modified Fe_3O_4@SiO_2 and VEGF shRNA or Notch-1 shRNA that had the property of gene silencing and magnetic resonance (MR) imaging [21]. Another study reported theencapsulation of 2 particles including DOX and two fluorescent materials comprising of FITC (fluores ceinisothiocyanate) and carbon quantum dots (C-dots) within chitosan nanoparticles having dual property of imaging and targeted therapy using VEGF shRNA nanoconjugates [22].

Another publication on chitosan that was PEGylated and targeted with folate ligand in gastric cancer demonstrated 5-FU/METHFR shRNA to deliver in multidrug resistance cells [23]. To reduce toxicity chitosan nanoparticles with gold nanoparticles were synthesized and delivered shRNAs to the human lungadenocarcinoma cells [24]. Gene silencing using shRNA was demonstrated of the voltage-gated K^+ channels was also achieved by the nanoconjugate as mentioned before [25]. To lower the cellular toxicity chitosan-graft-PEI (CHI---PEI) was used as an efficient gene carrier [26]. Moreover folate–chitosan-graf--PEI(FC-g-PEI) effectively targeted cancer cells and delivered shRNA. Akt1 shRNA delivery by this nanoconjugate demonstratedsuppression of lung tumorigenesis in mouse model [27]. Similarly, GFP tagged with this previously mentioned nanoconjugate showed excellent GFP expression in the lungs [28]. A new complex comprising of chitosan/protamine/shRNA are targeted to VEGF was found to be non-toxic with high transfection efficiency and gene silencing capability [29]. Chitosan in conjugation with tripolyphosphate (TPP) and shRNA was found to be highly efficient in transfection and biocompatible [30]. However, the use of transforming growth factor (TGFB1) shRNA in conjugation with the above nanoconjugate inhibited the epithelial cell proliferation [31]. In rhabdomyosarcomacells also this shRNA knocked down the protein synthesis

[32]. However, in another publication EGFR shRNA also demonstrated higher cellular in the cell line [33]. Another study showed low molecular weight chitosan (LMWC) as an efficient delivery vehicle of shRNA *in vitro* and *in vivo* [34]. VEGF shRNA-LMWC was found to suppress VEGF mRNA in tumor tissues with high bioavailability [35]. When anticancer druggefitinib and Atg-5 shRNAwas used they exhibited significant apoptosis, inhibits cytotoxicity and tumor growth *in vivo* [36]. Moreover, platelet-derived growth factor (PDGF) gene was also suppressed by the delivery of shRNAs in breast cancer cell lines. Further, Survivin shRNA and vascular endothelial growth factor (VEGF) siRNA was co-delivered by chitosan nanoparticle in conjugation with Galactose modified trimethylchitosan-cysteine (GTC) and showed synergistic treatment in hepatoma [37].

Another polymeric nanoparticle in solution is the dendrimers. They are highly branched polymeric molecules when they are in solution. One study demonstrated that dendrimer may be used for the delivery of pGL3 luciferase gene shRNA [38].

Poly(D,L-lactide-co-glycolide) (PLGA) nanoparticle is also a type of polymeric molecule. One of the largest shRNA of Annexin A2 gene was tried to deliver through the before said nanoparticle and it showed potential treatment efficiency in wide variety of disease conditions such as diabetic retinopathy, retinopathyfor prematurity, macular degenerationand cancer [39]. VEGF mRNAs were also suppressed by shRNAs delivered in conjugation with PLGA nanoparticle and demonstrated regression of corneal neovascularization [40]. When this PLGA is conjugated with JNK3-shRNA, they exhibited the inhibition of neural apoptosis in cerebral ischemia in oxygen and glucosedeprivation model (OGD model) [41]. In breast cancer cell line RAN gene was suppressed by shRNA in conjugation with PLGA and poly (ethylene glycol) (PEG) [42]. Not only in breast cancer but also in ovarian cancer also a study was conducted were focal adhesion kinase (FAK) and CD44 proteins were suppressed using shRNAs as both of them are overexpressed in ovarian cancer [43 - 46]. So the knockdown of these proteins helps in the inhibition of cancer growth, increasing the apoptosis,suppression of angiogenesis and reduced proliferation [47, 48].

Polyethylene glycol (PEG)is a type of polymeric nanoparticle that helped in the delivery of enhancer ofzeste homolog 2 (EZH2) shRNA in conjugation with a novel nanoconjugatemPEG-PEI that exhibited promising delivery in prostate cancer cell line [49]. Moreover, the co-delivery of living shRNA and surviving shRNA enhanced apoptosis and inhibited cell proliferation in PCa cells when they are delivered in conjugation with Monomethoxypolyethylene glycolchitosan (mPEG-CS) nanoparticles [50]. Another cancer *i.e.*, the ovarian cancer mouse model demonstrated decreased tumor growth when gro-α shRNA is delivered by follicle-stimulating hormone- peptide-conjugated PEG nanoparticle [51]. Another nanoconjugate was developed using follicle-stimulating hormone-Polyethylene glycol- Polyethyleneimine for the delivery of the same shRNA as mentioned before in ovarian cancer *in vivo* model [52]. In lung carcinoma cell line also a novel nanoparticle was used to deliver the BclxLshRNA [53].

Another type of polymeric nanoparticle is Polyethyleneimine (PEI). A nanoconjugate was formed using gold nanoparticle with chitosan-aconitic anhydride in conjugation with multidrug resistantgene ABCG2 shRNA to deliver it in liver cancer cells demonstrated greater efficiency [54]. In breast cancer *in vivo* and *in vitro* p65 shRNA was delivered that lead to anti-metastatic effect [55]. In another study same shRNA was used in conjugation with Tween 85-s-s-polyethyleneimine 2 K (TSP) that induced cellular apoptosis and inhibited cell proliferation, invasion in surrounding tissue [56]. In the same cancer model alkyl-modified polyethylenimine was used with PLGA to co-deliver Bcl-xLshRNA and DOX showed promising results [57]. In colon cancer *in vitro* model also demonstrated promising result on co-delivery of β-catenin and Bcl-2 shRNA in conjugation with PEI/chitosan-TBA nanoparticle [58]. CD44v6 shRNA was also delivered in the same cancer model in conjugation with PEG-PEI showed reduced the number of adenoma and growth [59]. To decrease the side effects of PEI another novel nanoconjugate was formulated using aptamer conjugated with PLL-alkyl-10%-PEI (PLPE8%) that delivered Bcl-XLshRNA and induced cellular apoptosis in breast cancer [60]. One more nanoconjugate was synthesized known as P85-PEI/TPGS/PTX/shSur complex nanoparticles(PTPNs) and this nanoconjugate delivered Paclitaxel (PTX) and surviving shRNA in lung cancer cell line [61]. In mouse colon adenocarcinoma the nanoconjugateAnti-KITENINshRNA-PEI-alt-PEG showed enhanced apoptosis and inhibited of cell proliferation *in vivo* [62]. In melanoma CXCR4-shRNA-jetPEInanoconjugate was used and this inhibited the pulmonary metastasis [63]. In prostate cancer combination therapy was used to deliver Bcl-xLshRNA and DOX that conjugated with aptamer-conjugated polyplexes [64]. Moreover, shRNA/PEI-PEG-APT/ DOX conjugate was also used as a part of combination therapy [65].

Other Nanoparticle Conjugates

Other than the above mentioned nanoparticles there are several other types of nanoconjugates that help in the treatment of the disease conditions. Survivin siRNA and adamantine-paclitaxel (Ada-PTX) was used for ovarian cancer therapy in conjugation with supramolecular micelles *i.e.*, PEI-CyD(PC) comprising of β-cyclodextrin (β-CyD) and polyethylenimine (PEI) [66]. In case of another types of cancer *i.e.*, prostate cancer was targeted using Androgen receptor(AR) shRNA in conjugation with H1 (folate-PEI600–cyclodextrin) nanopolymer for the treatment of hormone independent prostate cancer showed increased apoptosis and cell cycle arrest [67]. In case of malignantpleural mesothelioma (MPM) by anti-thymidylate synthase (TS) shRNA was used with a novel nanocarrier that helped to achieve greater clinical outcome [68]. In case of hypertension in rat model galactose linked Et to form Gal-PEG-Et (GPE) nanoparticle was conjugated with Angiotensinogen (AGT) shRNA was delivered and reduced blood pressure was achieved [69]. A new type of nanoconjugate was formulated using graphine oxide *i.e.*, GO–PEI–PEG/DOX/CS-Aco/PEI/shABCG2 and showed greater efficacy [70]. A nanoconjugate was fabricated using single-walled carbon nanotubes(SWCNTs) covalently attached PEG and PEI that delivered Bcl-xLshRNA in breast cancer cell lines [71]. Moreover, gold nanorods were also used to deliver luciferase shRNA and opened a new avenue of gene delivery [72]. EGFP shRNA was also delivered and a comparison was studies using three novel poly (β-amine esters) (PAEs) that have differentamino monomers in the main chain and gene silencing was achieved *in vitro* and *in vivo* [73]. For myocardial fibrosis treatment Connective tissue growth factor (CTGF) shRNA was loaded in PAMAM and proved to be effective [74]. A new delivery vehicle poly(2-dimethyl amino ethylamine /2-(2-amino ethyoxy) ethoxy) phos phazene (PDMAE) was used to deliver surviving shRNA in breast cancer showed a potent delivery vehicle for chemotherapy [75]. Another major variety of use of shRNAs are the use of bi-shRNAs such as pancreaticand duodenal homeobox 1shRNA was used in conjugation with bilamell arinvaginat edvesicles (BIV) and are in the phase I trial [76]. In case of lung cancer also Akt1shRNA in conjugation with poly(b-amino ester) (PAE) showed greater efficacy in comparison with PEI25K nanoparticle [77]. Protaminenanoparticle was also fabricated to knockdown Bcl-2 gene in a study [78]. Excellent tumor icidaleffect was demonstrated in a nanoconjugated that was fabricated using single-walled carbon nano tubes polyethyleneglycol-polyethylenimine (SWNT-PEG-PEI) attached with AS1411 aptamer and Bcl-xL-specific shRNA for targeting gastric cancer cells [79]. TRITC-gene regulation nanoparticles (GRN) nanoparticle when complexed with RUNX2, SOX9, pDNA, shATF4, ATF4, pDNAs, and C/EBPα pDNA they are found to have higher expression of adipogenesis, osteogenesisand chondrogenesis [80]. MDR breast cancer was also treated effectively using Core shell poly lactide (PLA) when they are co-delivered with DOX and multi drug resistance protein 1 (MDR1) targeted shRNAs (Table **1**) [81].

Table 1. shRNA nanoparticles conjugate with their target gene and diseases.

Nanoparticle	Disease	Target Gene	References
Chitosan	Cancer	VEGF, Notch-1, METHFR, GFP, TGFB1, EGFR, Atg-5,PDG--D,Survivin	[22-25, 33, 36, 82-89]

(Table 1) cont.....

Nanoparticle	Disease	Target Gene	References
Dendrimer	Cancer	pGL3 luciferase	[38]
Gold	Cancer	p53, MCL-1, LRP5	[7, 90]
Lipid	Hepatitis C	IRES	[91, 92]
lipid	Cancer	p5α-Red, CLDN3, FRα, EWS/FLI1	[20, 93, 94]
PLGA	diabetic retinopathy, retinopathy for prematurity, cancer and macular degeneration	Annexin A2	[39]
PLGA	corneal neovascularization	VEGF-A	[95]
PLGA	OGD model	JNK3	[41]
PLGA	Cancer	RAN, FAK, CD44	[48, 96-98]
PEI	Cancer	ABCG2, p65, Bcl-xL, β-catenin, Bcl-2, CD44v6, surviving, KITENIN, CXCR4, Bcl-xL, PSMA, DNAPK	[54, 56-58, 61-63, 99-106]
Magnetic nanoparticle	Cancer	SATB1, MDR1, IGF-1R, pHSP70-Plk1	[9, 11, 12]
Magnetic nanoparticle	Parkinson's disease	α-synuclein	[107]
PEG	Cancer	EZH2, livin, surviving, gro-α, Bcl-xL	[108-112]
Silica nanoparticle	Cancer	Surviving, p-gp	[15, 113]
Other nanoparticles	Cancer	Surviving, AR, TS, ABCG2, Bcl-xL, luciferase, EGFP, PDX1, Akt1, Bcl-2, MDR1	[67, 68, 70, 72, 76, 78, 81, 114-119]
Other nanoparticles	Hypertension	AGT	[69]
Other nanoparticles	Myocardial fibrosis	CTGF	[74]
Other nanoparticles	Osteogenesis	ATF4	[80]

CONCLUSION

In the area of shRNA-nanoparticle conjugate delivery, there are several challenges that should be addressed before their clinical application. The hurdles that are faced by the researchers in this application are the off-target toxicity [120]. The nanoconjugate should be targeted specifically to the site where the suppression of genetic expression is needed [121]. Many phase I and phase II trials are going on such as Gradalis Inc. (Carrollton, Texas, USA) is conducting phaseI and II trials for ovarian cancer using FANG™ Vaccine that expresses both Furinbi functional shRNAs [122]. Another such trial is being conducted by Marina Biotech (Bothell, Washington, USA; formerly CequentPharmaceuticals) using β-catenin shRNA for the treatment of Familial Adenomatous Polyposis (FAP) [123].

The bare shRNAs have several hurdles in their application as they are highly fragile molecules and they readily degrade in the blood by the enzymatic actions. In this aspect, nanoparticles have a definite role to play as they encapsulate the nanoconjugate and protect them from degradation in the blood stream. Selection of particular nanoconjugate depends on the property of the nanoplatform, based on the route of administration, nature of active moiety, site of action, and fabrication techniques. Biocompatible inorganic, organic or hybrid nanomaterials are preferred for better efficacy, low toxicity and low antigenic response by accumulation for longer duration. The clinical trials are facing many hurdles in these respects, although the researches have made shRNA-nanoparticle conjugate a potential therapeutic option for many diseases conditions.

REFERENCES

[1] Aagaard L, Rossi JJ. RNAi therapeutics: principles, prospects and challenges. Adv Drug Deliv Rev 2007; 59(2-3): 75-86.
[http://dx.doi.org/10.1016/j.addr.2007.03.005] [PMID: 17449137]

[2] Moore CB, Guthrie EH, Huang MT, Taxman DJ. Short hairpin RNA (shRNA): design, delivery, and assessment of gene knockdown. Methods Mol Biol 2010; 629: 141-58.
[PMID: 20387148]

[3] Acharya R. The recent progresses in shRNA-nanoparticle conjugate as a therapeutic approach. Mater Sci Eng C 2019; 104: 109928.
[http://dx.doi.org/10.1016/j.msec.2019.109928]

[4] Ovcharenko D, Jarvis R, Hunicke-Smith S, Kelnar K, Brown D. High-throughput RNAi screening *in vitro*: from cell lines to primary cells. RNA 2005; 11(6): 985-93.
[http://dx.doi.org/10.1261/rna.7288405] [PMID: 15923380]

[5] Dyer V, Ely A, Bloom K, Weinberg M, Arbuthnot P. tRNA Lys3 promoter cassettes that efficiently express RNAi-activating antihepatitis B virus short hairpin RNAs. Biochem Biophys Res Commun 2010; 398(4): 640-6.
[http://dx.doi.org/10.1016/j.bbrc.2010.06.122] [PMID: 20599752]

[6] Acharya R, Saha S, Ray S, Hazra S, Mitra MK, Chakraborty J. siRNA-nanoparticle conjugate in gene silencing: A future cure to deadly diseases? Mater Sci Eng C 2017; 76: 1378-400.
[http://dx.doi.org/10.1016/j.msec.2017.03.009] [PMID: 28482505]

[7] Ryou S-M, Kim S, Jang HH, Kim J-H, Yeom J-H, Eom MS, *et al.* Delivery of shRNA using gold nanoparticle–DNA oligonucleotide conjugates as a universal carrier. Biochem Biophys Res Commun 2010; 398(3): 542-6.
[http://dx.doi.org/10.1016/j.bbrc.2010.06.115]

[8] Li C, Li Z, Zhang Y, Fathy AH, Zhou M. The role of the Wnt/β-catenin signaling pathway in the proliferation of gold nanoparticle-treated human periodontal ligament stem cells. Stem Cell Res Ther 2018; 9(1): 214. http://europepmc.org/abstract/MED/30092818

[9] Peng Z, Wang C, Fang E, Lu X, Wang G, Tong Q. Co-delivery of doxorubicin and SATB1 shRNA by thermosensitive magnetic cationic liposomes for gastric cancer therapy. PLoS One 2014; 9(3): e92924.
[http://dx.doi.org/10.1371/journal.pone.0092924] [PMID: 24675979]

[10] Chen BA, Mao PP, Cheng J, *et al.* Reversal of multidrug resistance by magnetic Fe3O4 nanoparticle copolymerizating daunorubicin and MDR1 shRNA expression vector in leukemia cells. Int J Nanomedicine 2010; 5: 437-44.
[http://dx.doi.org/10.2147/IJN.S10083] [PMID: 20957165]

[11] Kong M, Li X, Wang C, *et al.* Tissue distribution and cancer growth inhibition of magnetic lipoplex-delivered type 1 insulin-like growth factor receptor shRNA in nude mice. Acta Biochim Biophys Sin (Shanghai) 2012; 44(7): 591-6.
[http://dx.doi.org/10.1093/abbs/gms039] [PMID: 22626974]

[12] Cheng L, Ke Y, Yu S, Jing J. Co-delivery of doxorubicin and recombinant plasmid pHSP70-Plk--shRNA by bacterial magnetosomes for osteosarcoma therapy. Int J Nanomedicine 2016; 11: 5277-86.
[http://dx.doi.org/10.2147/IJN.S115364] [PMID: 27822032]

[13] Niu S, Zhang L-K, Zhang L, *et al.* Inhibition by multifunctional magnetic nanoparticles loaded with alpha-synuclein RNAi plasmid in a Parkinson's disease model. Theranostics 2017; 7(2): 344-56.
[http://dx.doi.org/10.7150/thno.16562] [PMID: 28042339]

[14] Li Z, Zhang L, Tang C, Yin C. Co-delivery of doxorubicin and survivin shRNA-expressing plasmid *via* microenvironment-responsive dendritic mesoporous silica nanoparticles for synergistic cancer therapy. Pharm Res 2017; 34(12): 2829-41.
[http://dx.doi.org/10.1007/s11095-017-2264-6] [PMID: 28948461]

[15] Yang H, Chen Y, Chen Z, *et al.* Chemo-photodynamic combined gene therapy and dual-modal cancer imaging achieved by pH-responsive alginate/chitosan multilayer-modified magnetic mesoporous silica nanocomposites. Biomater Sci 2017; 5(5): 1001-13.
[http://dx.doi.org/10.1039/C7BM00043J] [PMID: 28327716]

[16] Torrecilla J, del Pozo-Rodríguez A, Apaolaza PS, Solinís MÁ, Rodríguez-Gascón A. Solid lipid nanoparticles as non-viral vector for the treatment of chronic hepatitis C by RNA interference. Int J Pharm 2015; 479(1): 181-8.
[http://dx.doi.org/10.1016/j.ijpharm.2014.12.047] [PMID: 25542984]

[17] Akbaba H, Erel Akbaba G, Kantarci A. Development and evaluation of antisense shRNA-encoding plasmid loaded solid lipid nanoparticles against 5-α reductase activity. J Drug Deliv Sci Technol 2018; 01(01): 44.
[http://dx.doi.org/10.1016/j.jddst.2018.01.001]

[18] Dallas A, Ilves H, Shorenstein J, Judge A, Spitler R, Contag C, *et al.* Minimal-length synthetic shRNAs formulated with lipid nanoparticles are potent inhibitors of hepatitis C virus IRES-linked gene expression in mice. Mol Therapy Nucleic Acids 2013: e123.

[19] He ZY, Wei XW, Luo M, Luo ST, Yang Y, Yu YY, *et al.* Folate-linked lipoplexes for short hairpin RNA targeting claudin-3 delivery in ovarian cancer xenografts. J Control Rel: Off. J Control Rel Soc 2013; 172(3): 679-89.
[PMID: 24144916] [http://dx.doi.org/10.1016/j.jconrel.2013.10.015]

[20] Rao DD, Jay C, Wang Z, Luo X, Kumar P, Eysenbach H, *et al.* Preclinical Justification of pbi-shRNA EWS/FLI1 Lipoplex (LPX) Treatment for Ewing's Sarcoma. Molecular therapy: J American Soc of Gene Therapy 2016; 24(8): 1412-22.
[PMID: 27166877]

[21] Li T, Shen X, Chen Y, *et al.* Polyetherimide-grafted $Fe_3O_6@SiO_2$ nanoparticles as theranostic agents for simultaneous VEGF siRNA delivery and magnetic resonance cell imaging. Int J Nanomedicine 2015; 10: 4279-91.
[http://dx.doi.org/10.2147/IJN.S85095] [PMID: 26170664]

[22] Yang H, Xu M, Li S, Shen X, Li T, Yan J, *et al.* Chitosan hybrid nanoparticles as a theranostic platform for targeted doxorubicin/VEGF shRNA co-delivery and dual-modality fluorescence imaging. RSC Advances 2016; 6(35): 29685-96.
[http://dx.doi.org/10.1039/C6RA03843C]

[23] Xin L, Fan J-C, Le Y-G, Zeng F, Cheng H, Hu X-y, *et al.* Construction of METHFR shRNA/5-fluorouracil co-loaded folate-targeted chitosan polymeric nanoparticles and its anti-carcinoma effect on gastric cells growth. J Nanopart Res 2016; 18(5): 105.

[24] Jeong S, Choi SY, Park J, Seo J-H, Park J, Cho K, *et al.* Low-toxicity chitosan gold nanoparticles for small hairpin RNA delivery in human lung adenocarcinoma cells. J Mater Chem 2011; 21(36): 13853-9.
[http://dx.doi.org/10.1039/c1jm11913c]

[25] Jang SH, Choi SY, Ryu PD, Lee SY. Anti-proliferative effect of Kv1.3 blockers in A549 human lung adenocarcinoma *in vitro* and *in vivo*. European J Pharm 2011; 651(1): 26-32.

[26] Jiang H-L, Kim Y-K, Arote R, Nah J-W, Cho M-H, Choi Y-J, *et al.* Chitosan-graft-polyethylenimine as a gene carrier. J Cont Rel 2007; 117(2): 273-80.
[http://dx.doi.org/10.1016/j.jconrel.2006.10.025]

[27] Gautam A, Clifford Waldrep J, Densmore CL. Aerosol gene therapy. Molecular Biotechnology 2003; 23(1): 51-60.
[http://dx.doi.org/10.1385/MB:23:1:51]

[28] Jiang HL, Xu CX, Kim YK, *et al.* The suppression of lung tumorigenesis by aerosol-delivered folate-chitosan-graft-polyethylenimine/Akt1 shRNA complexes through the Akt signaling pathway. Biomaterials 2009; 30(29): 5844-52.
[http://dx.doi.org/10.1016/j.biomaterials.2009.07.017] [PMID: 19640582]

[29] Erdem-Çakmak F, Özbaş-Turan S, Şalva E, Akbuğa J. Comparison of VEGF gene silencing efficiencies of chitosan and protamine complexes containing shRNA. Cell Biol Int 2014; 38(11): 1260-70.
[http://dx.doi.org/10.1002/cbin.10317] [PMID: 24890139]

[30] López-León T, Carvalho EL, Seijo B, Ortega-Vinuesa JL, Bastos-González D. Physicochemical characterization of chitosan nanoparticles: electrokinetic and stability behavior. J Colloid Interface Sci 2005; 283(2): 344-51.
[http://dx.doi.org/10.1016/j.jcis.2004.08.186] [PMID: 15721903]

[31] Roberts AB, Wakefield LM. The two faces of transforming growth factor β in carcinogenesis. Proc Natl Acad Sci USA 2003; 100(15): 8621-3.
[http://dx.doi.org/10.1073/pnas.1633291100] [PMID: 12861075]

[32] Wang SL, Yao HH, Guo LL, *et al.* Selection of optimal sites for TGFB1 gene silencing by chitosan-TPP nanoparticle-mediated delivery of shRNA. Cancer Genet Cytogenet 2009; 190(1): 8-14.
[http://dx.doi.org/10.1016/j.cancergencyto.2008.10.013] [PMID: 19264227]

[33] Karimi M, Avci P, Ahi M, Gazori T, Hamblin MR, Naderi-Manesh H. Evaluation of Chitosan-Tripolyphosphate Nanoparticles as a p-shRNA Delivery Vector: Formulation, Optimization and Cellular Uptake Study. J Nanopharm Drug Deliv. 2013; 1(3): 266-78.
[PMID: 26989641]

[34] Petros RA, DeSimone JM. Strategies in the design of nanoparticles for therapeutic applications. Nat Rev Drug Discov 2010; 9(8): 615-27.
[http://dx.doi.org/10.1038/nrd2591]

[35] Huang Z, Dong L, Chen J, *et al.* Low-molecular weight chitosan/vascular endothelial growth factor short hairpin RNA for the treatment of hepatocellular carcinoma. Life Sci 2012; 91(23-24): 1207-15.
[http://dx.doi.org/10.1016/j.lfs.2012.09.015] [PMID: 23044224]

[36] Zheng Y, Su C, Zhao L, Shi Y. Chitosan nanoparticle-mediated co-delivery of shAtg-5 and gefitinib synergistically promoted the efficacy of chemotherapeutics through the modulation of autophagy. J Nanobiotechnol 2017; 15(1): 28.
[http://dx.doi.org/10.1186/s12951-017-0261-x]

[37] Han L, Tang C, Yin C. Oral delivery of shRNA and siRNA *via* multifunctional polymeric

nanoparticles for synergistic cancer therapy. Biomaterials 2014; 35(15): 4589-600. [http://dx.doi.org/10.1016/j.biomaterials.2014.02.027] [PMID: 24613049]

[38] Arima H, Motoyama K, Higashi T. Polyamidoamine dendrimer conjugates with cyclodextrins as novel carriers for DNA, shRNA and siRNA. Pharmaceutics 2012; 4(1): 130-48. [http://dx.doi.org/10.3390/pharmaceutics4010130] [PMID: 24300184]

[39] Mukerjee A, Shankardas J, Ranjan AP, Vishwanatha JK. Efficient nanoparticle mediated sustained RNA interference in human primary endothelial cells. Nanotechnology 2011; 22(44): 445101. [http://dx.doi.org/10.1088/0957-4484/22/44/445101] [PMID: 21990205]

[40] Qazi Y, Stagg B, Singh N, Singh S, Zhang X, Luo L, *et al.* Nanoparticle-mediated delivery of shRNA.VEGF-a plasmids regresses corneal neovascularization. Investigative Ophthalmology and Visual Science 2012; 53(6): 2837-44. [PMID: 22467572]

[41] Zheng J, Qi J, Zou Q, Zhang Z. Construction of PLGA/JNK3-shRNA nanoparticles and their protective role in hippocampal neuron apoptosis induced by oxygen and glucose deprivation. RSC Advances 2018; 8(36): 20108-16. [http://dx.doi.org/10.1039/C8RA00679B]

[42] Sharma A, McCarron P, Matchett K, Hawthorne S, El-Tanani M. Anti-invasive and anti-proliferative effects of shrna-loaded poly (Lactide-Co-Glycolide) Nanoparticles Following RAN Silencing in MDA-MB231 Breast Cancer Cells. Pharm Res 2018; 36(2): 26.

[43] Sood AK, Coffin JE, Schneider GB, *et al.* Biological significance of focal adhesion kinase in ovarian cancer: role in migration and invasion. Am J Pathol 2004; 165(4): 1087-95. [http://dx.doi.org/10.1016/S0002-9440(10)63370-6] [PMID: 15466376]

[44] Shen T-L, Park AYJ, Alcaraz A, *et al.* Conditional knockout of focal adhesion kinase in endothelial cells reveals its role in angiogenesis and vascular development in late embryogenesis. J Cell Biol 2005; 169(6): 941-52. [http://dx.doi.org/10.1083/jcb.200411155] [PMID: 15967814]

[45] Sleeman J, Rudy W, Hofmann M, Moll J, Herrlich P, Ponta H. Regulated clustering of variant CD44 proteins increases their hyaluronate binding capacity. J Cell Biol 1996; 135(4): 1139-50. [http://dx.doi.org/10.1083/jcb.135.4.1139] [PMID: 8922392]

[46] Ponta H, Wainwright D, Herrlich P. The CD44 protein family. Int J Biochem Cell Biol 1998; 30(3): 299-305. [http://dx.doi.org/10.1016/S1357-2725(97)00152-0] [PMID: 9611772]

[47] Halder J, Kamat AA, Landen CN, Han LY, Lutgendorf SK, Lin YG, *et al.* Focal adhesion kinase targeting using *in vivo* short interfering RNA delivery in neutral liposomes for ovarian carcinoma therapy. Clin Cancer Res 2006; 12(16): 4916-24. [http://dx.doi.org/10.1158/1078-0432.CCR-06-0021] [PMID: 16914580]

[48] Bapat SA, Mali AM, Koppikar CB, Kurrey NK. Stem and progenitor-like cells contribute to the aggressive behavior of human epithelial ovarian cancer. Cancer Res 2005; 65(8): 3025-9. [http://dx.doi.org/10.1158/0008-5472.CAN-04-3931] [PMID: 15833827]

[49] Wu Y, Yu J, Liu Y, *et al.* Delivery of EZH2-shRNA with mPEG-PEI nanoparticles for the treatment of prostate cancer *in vitro*. Int J Mol Med 2014; 33(6): 1563-9. [http://dx.doi.org/10.3892/ijmm.2014.1724] [PMID: 24714818]

[50] Huang Q, Zeng Y, Lin H, Zhang H, Yang D. Transfection with livin and survivin shRNA inhibits the growth and proliferation of non□small cell lung cancer cells. Mol Med Rep 2017; 16(5): 7086-91. [http://dx.doi.org/10.3892/mmr.2017.7490] [PMID: 28901499]

[51] Zhang M-X, Hong S-S, Cai Q-Q, Zhang M, Chen J, Zhang X-Y, *et al.* Transcriptional control of the MUC16 promoter facilitates follicle-stimulating hormone peptide-conjugated shRNA nanoparticle-mediated inhibition of ovarian carcinoma *in vivo*. Drug Delivery 2018; 25(1): 797-806.

[http://dx.doi.org/10.1080/10717544.2018.1451934]

[52] Hong S-S, Zhang M-X, Zhang M, Yu Y, Chen J, Zhang X-Y, *et al.* Follicle-stimulating hormone peptide-conjugated nanoparticles for targeted shRNA delivery lead to effective gro-α silencing and antitumor activity against ovarian cancer. Drug Delivery 2018; 25(1): 576-84. [http://dx.doi.org/10.1080/10717544.2018.1440667]

[53] Ayatollahi S, Salmasi Z, Hashemi M, *et al.* Aptamer-targeted delivery of Bcl-xL shRNA using alkyl modified PAMAM dendrimers into lung cancer cells. Int J Biochem Cell Biol 2017; 92: 210-7. [http://dx.doi.org/10.1016/j.biocel.2017.10.005] [PMID: 29031805]

[54] Chen Z, Zhang L, He Y, Shen Y, Li Y. Enhanced shRNA delivery and abcg2 silencing by charge-reversible layered nanocarriers. Small 2015; 11(8): 952-62. [http://dx.doi.org/10.1002/smll.201401397]

[55] Xiao J, Duan X, Meng Q, *et al.* Effective delivery of p65 shRNA by optimized Tween 85-polyethyleneimine conjugate for inhibition of tumor growth and lymphatic metastasis. Acta Biomater 2014; 10(6): 2674-83. [http://dx.doi.org/10.1016/j.actbio.2014.02.009] [PMID: 24525035]

[56] Xiao J, Duan X, Yin Q, Miao Z, Yu H, Chen C, *et al.* The inhibition of metastasis and growth of breast cancer by blocking the NF-κB signaling pathway using bioreducible PEI-based/p65 shRNA complex nanoparticles. Biomaterials 2013; 34(21): 5381-90.

[57] Ebrahimian M, Taghavi S, Mokhtarzadeh A, Ramezani M, Hashemi M. Co-delivery of doxorubicin encapsulated PLGA nanoparticles and Bcl-xL shRNA using alkyl-modified PEI into Breast Cancer Cells. App Biochem Biotechn 2017; 183(1): 126-36. [http://dx.doi.org/10.1007/s12010-017-2434-3]

[58] Javan B, Atyabi F, Shahbazi M. Hypoxia-inducible bidirectional shRNA expression vector delivery using PEI/chitosan-TBA copolymers for colorectal Cancer gene therapy. Life Sci 2018; 202: 140-51.

[59] Misra S, Hascall VC, De Giovanni C, Markwald RR, Ghatak S. Delivery of CD44 shRNA/nanoparticles within cancer cells: perturbation of hyaluronan/CD44v6 interactions and reduction in adenoma growth in Apc Min/+ MICE. J Biol Chem 2009; 284(18): 12432-46. [http://dx.doi.org/10.1074/jbc.M806772200] [PMID: 19246453]

[60] Askarian S, Abnous K, Taghavi S, Oskuee RK, Ramezani M. Cellular delivery of shRNA using aptamer-conjugated PLL-alkyl-PEI nanoparticles. Colloids Surf B Biointerfaces 2015; 136: 355-64. [PMID: 26433348]

[61] Shen J, Yin Q, Chen L, Zhang Z, Li Y. Co-delivery of paclitaxel and survivin shRNA by pluronic P85-PEI/TPGS complex nanoparticles to overcome drug resistance in lung cancer. Biomaterials 2012; 33(33): 8613-24.

[62] Park IK, Kim KK, Cho SH, *et al.* Intratumoral administration of anti-KITENIN shRNA-loaded PEI-alt-PEG nanoparticles suppressed colon carcinoma established subcutaneously in mice. J Nanosci Nanotechnol 2010; 10(5): 3280-3. [http://dx.doi.org/10.1166/jnn.2010.2231] [PMID: 20358939]

[63] André ND, Silva VA, Ariza CB, Watanabe MA, De Lucca FL. In vivo knockdown of CXCR4 using jetPEI/CXCR4 shRNA nanoparticles inhibits the pulmonary metastatic potential of B16-F10 melanoma cells. Mol Med Rep 2015; 12(6): 8320-6. [http://dx.doi.org/10.3892/mmr.2015.4487] [PMID: 26498029]

[64] Lupold SE, Hicke BJ, Lin Y, Coffey DS. Identification and characterization of nuclease-stabilized RNA molecules that bind human prostate cancer cells via the prostate-specific membrane antigen. Cancer Res 2002; 62(14): 4029-33. [PMID: 12124337]

[65] Kim E, Jung Y, Choi H, Yang J, Suh J-S, Huh Y-M, *et al.* Prostate cancer cell death produced by the co-delivery of Bcl-xL shRNA and doxorubicin using an aptamer-conjugated polyplex. Biomaterials

2010; 31(16): 4592-9.
[http://dx.doi.org/10.1016/j.biomaterials.2010.02.030] [PMID: 20206379]

[66] Hu Q, Li W, Hu X, *et al.* Synergistic treatment of ovarian cancer by co-delivery of survivin shRNA and paclitaxel *via* supramolecular micellar assembly. Biomaterials 2012; 33(27): 6580-91. [http://dx.doi.org/10.1016/j.biomaterials.2012.05.060] [PMID: 22717365]

[67] Zhang X, Liu N, Shao Z, Qiu H, Yao H, Ji J, *et al.* Folate-targeted nanoparticle delivery of androgen receptor shRNA enhances the sensitivity of hormone-independent prostate cancer to radiotherapy. Nanomedicine: Nanotechnology, Biology and Medicine 2017; 13(4): 1309-21. [http://dx.doi.org/10.1016/j.nano.2017.01.015]

[68] Ishida T, Abu Lila A, Huang C, Wada H, Fukushima M, Kiwada H. 230 an entirely novel nanoparticle carrying a bioactive shRNA molecule (DFP-10825) could be clinically effective against the high risk patients with mesothelioma relapsed or refractory after treatment with pemetrexed based chemotherapy. Eur J Canc 2012; 48: 69-70.

[69] Lu P, Yuan L, Wang Y, Du Q, Sheng J. Effect of GPE-AGT nanoparticle shRNA transfection system mediated RNAi on early atherosclerotic lesion. Int J Clin Exp Pathol 2012; 5(7): 698-706. [PMID: 22977667]

[70] He Y, Zhang L, Chen Z, *et al.* Enhanced chemotherapy efficacy by co-delivery of shABCG2 and doxorubicin with a pH-responsive charge-reversible layered graphene oxide nanocomplex. J Mater Chem B Mater Biol Med 2015; 3(31): 6462-72. [http://dx.doi.org/10.1039/C5TB00923E] [PMID: 32262554]

[71] Dizaji BF, Farboudi A, Rahbar A, Azarbaijan MH, Asgary MR. The role of single- and multi-walled carbon nanotube in breast cancer treatment. Ther Deliv 2020; 11(10): 653-72. [http://dx.doi.org/10.4155/tde-2020-0019] [PMID: 32475258]

[72] Ramos J, Rege K. Poly (aminoether)–gold nanorod assemblies for shRNA plasmid-induced gene silencing. Mol Pharm 2013; 10(11): 4107-19.

[73] Yin Q, Gao Y, Zhang Z, Zhang P, Li Y. Bioreducible poly (β-amino esters)/shRNA complex nanoparticles for efficient RNA delivery. J Control Rel Soc 2011; 151(1): 35-44. [PMID: 21244853]

[74] Huang ZJ, Yi B, Yuan H, Yang GP. Efficient delivery of connective tissue growth factor shRNA using PAMAM nanoparticles. Genet Mol Res 2014; 13(3): 6716-23. [http://dx.doi.org/10.4238/2014.August.28.15] [PMID: 25177951]

[75] Yang Y, Gao Y, Chen L, Huang Y, Li Y. Downregulation of survivin expression and enhanced chemosensitivity of MCF-7 cells to adriamycin by PDMAE/survivin shRNA complex nanoparticles. Int J Pharm 2011; 405(1-2): 188-95. [http://dx.doi.org/10.1016/j.ijpharm.2010.11.047] [PMID: 21130850]

[76] Jay CM, Ruoff C, Kumar P, Maass H, Spanhel B, Miller M, *et al.* Assessment of intravenous pbi-shRNA PDX1 nanoparticle (OFHIRNA-PDX1) in yucatan swine. Canc Gene Ther 2013; 20(12): 683-9.

[77] Jere D, Xu CX, Arote R, Yun CH, Cho MH, Cho CS. Poly(beta-amino ester) as a carrier for si/shRNA delivery in lung cancer cells. Biomaterials 2008; 29(16): 2535-47. [http://dx.doi.org/10.1016/j.biomaterials.2008.02.018] [PMID: 18316120]

[78] Liu M, Feng B, Shi Y, Su C, Song H, Cheng W, *et al.* Protamine nanoparticles for improving shRNA-mediated anti-cancer effects. Nanoscale Res Letters 2015; 10(1):134. [http://dx.doi.org/10.1186/s11671-015-0845-z]

[79] Taghavi S, Nia AH, Abnous K, Ramezani M. Polyethylenimine-functionalized carbon nanotubes tagged with AS1411 aptamer for combination gene and drug delivery into human gastric cancer cells. Intern J Pharmaceu 2017; 516(1-2): 301-12. [http://dx.doi.org/10.1016/j.ijpharm.2016.11.027] [PMID: 27840158]

[80] Kim HJ, Yi SW, Oh HJ, Lee JS, Park JS, Park K-H. Transfection of gene regulation nanoparticles complexed with pDNA and shRNA controls multilineage differentiation of hMSCs. Biomater 2018; 177: 1-13.
[http://dx.doi.org/10.1016/j.biomaterials.2018.05.035] [PMID: 29883913]

[81] Ni Q, Zhang F, Zhang Y, Zhu G, Wang Z, Teng Z, *et al. In Situ* shRNA synthesis on DNA–Polylactide nanoparticles to treat multidrug resistant breast cancer. Adv Mater 2018; 30(10): 1705737.

[82] Jiang H-L, Xu C-X, Kim Y-K, Arote R, Jere D, Lim H-T, *et al.* The suppression of lung tumorigenesis by aerosol-delivered folate–chitosan-graft-polyethylenimine/Akt1 shRNA complexes through the Akt signaling pathway. Biomater 2009; 30(29): 5844-52.

[83] Erdem-Çakmak F, Özbaş-Turan S, Şalva E, Akbuğa J. Comparison of VEGF gene silencing efficiencies of chitosan and protamine complexes containing shRNA. Cell Biol Int 2014; 38(11): 1260-70.
[http://dx.doi.org/10.1002/cbin.10317] [PMID: 24890139]

[84] Wang S-L, Yao H-H, Guo L-L, Dong L, Li S-G, Gu Y-P, *et al.* Selection of optimal sites for TGFB1 gene silencing by chitosan–TPP nanoparticle-mediated delivery of shRNA. Cancer Genetics and Cytogenetics 2009; 190(1): 8-14.
[http://dx.doi.org/10.1016/j.cancergencyto.2008.10.013]

[85] Kim SH, Jeong JH, Lee SH, Kim SW, Park TG. Local and systemic delivery of VEGF siRNA using polyelectrolyte complex micelles for effective treatment of cancer. J Control Rel 2008; 129(2): 107-16.
[http://dx.doi.org/10.1016/j.jconrel.2008.03.008]

[86] Takei Y, Kadomatsu K, Yuzawa Y, Matsuo S, Muramatsu T. A small interfering RNA targeting vascular endothelial growth factor as cancer therapeutics. Cancer Res 2004; 64(10): 3365-70.
[http://dx.doi.org/10.1158/0008-5472.CAN-03-2682] [PMID: 15150085]

[87] Huang Z, Dong L, Chen J, Gao F, Zhang Z, Chen J, *et al.* Low-molecular weight chitosan/vascular endothelial growth factor short hairpin RNA for the treatment of hepatocellular carcinoma. Life Sci 2012; 91(23): 1207-15.

[88] Özbaş-Turan S, Akbuga J, Ekentok C. *In vitro* gene silencing effect of chitosan/shRNA PDGF-D nanoparticles in breast cancer. Marmara Pharmaceutical J 2017; 21: 793-803.

[89] Han L, Tang C, Yin C. Oral delivery of shRNA and siRNA via multifunctional polymeric nanoparticles for synergistic cancer therapy. Biomater 2014; 35(15): 4589-600.
[http://dx.doi.org/10.1016/j.biomaterials.2014.02.027]

[90] Li C, Li Z, Zhang Y, Fathy AH, Zhou M. The role of the Wnt/β-catenin signaling pathway in the proliferation of gold nanoparticle-treated human periodontal ligament stem cells. Stem Cell Res Ther 2018; 9(1): 214.

[91] Torrecilla J, del Pozo-Rodríguez A, Apaolaza PS, Solinís MÁ, Rodríguez-Gascón A. Solid lipid nanoparticles as non-viral vector for the treatment of chronic hepatitis C by RNA interference. Intern J Pharma 2015; 479(1): 181-8.
[http://dx.doi.org/10.1016/j.ijpharm.2014.12.047]

[92] Dallas A, Ilves H, Shorenstein J, *et al.* Minimal-length Synthetic shRNAs Formulated with Lipid Nanoparticles are Potent Inhibitors of Hepatitis C Virus IRES-linked Gene Expression in Mice. Mol Ther Nucleic Acids 2013; 2(9): e123.
[http://dx.doi.org/10.1038/mtna.2013.50] [PMID: 24045712]

[93] Akbaba H, Erel Akbaba G, Kantarcı AG. Development and evaluation of antisense shRNA-encoding plasmid loaded solid lipid nanoparticles against 5-α reductase activity. J Drug Del Sci Techn 2018; 44: 270-7.

[94] He Z-Y, Wei X-W, Luo M, Luo S-T, Yang Y, Yu Y-Y, *et al.* Folate-linked lipoplexes for short hairpin

RNA targeting claudin-3 delivery in ovarian cancer xenografts. J Control Rel 2013; 172(3): 679-89. [http://dx.doi.org/10.1016/j.jconrel.2013.10.015]

[95] Qazi Y, Stagg B, Singh N, *et al.* Nanoparticle-mediated delivery of shRNA.VEGF-a plasmids regresses corneal neovascularization. Invest Ophthalmol Vis Sci 2012; 53(6): 2837-44. [http://dx.doi.org/10.1167/iovs.11-9139] [PMID: 22467572]

[96] Sharma A, Hawthorne S, El-Tanani M, McCarron P. *In-vitro* evaluation of shRNA Nanoparticles for anti-metastasis RanGTPase Biotherapeutics 2015.

[97] Halder J, Kamat AA, Landen CN Jr, *et al.* Focal adhesion kinase targeting using in vivo short interfering RNA delivery in neutral liposomes for ovarian carcinoma therapy. Clin Cancer Res 2006; 12(16): 4916-24. [http://dx.doi.org/10.1158/1078-0432.CCR-06-0021] [PMID: 16914580]

[98] Zou L, Song X, Yi T, Li S, Deng H, Chen X, *et al.* Administration of PLGA nanoparticles carrying shRNA against focal adhesion kinase and CD44 results in enhanced antitumor effects against ovarian cancer. Cancer Gene Therapy 2013; 20(4): 242-50. [http://dx.doi.org/10.1038/cgt.2013.12]

[99] Xiao J, Duan X, Meng Q, Yin Q, Zhang Z, Yu H, *et al.* Effective delivery of p65 shRNA by optimized Tween 85-polyethyleneimine conjugate for inhibition of tumor growth and lymphatic metastasis. Acta biomater 2014; 10(6): 2674-83.

[100] Misra S, Hascall VC, De Giovanni C, Markwald RR, Ghatak S. Delivery of CD44 shRNA/nanoparticles within cancer cells: perturbation of hyaluronan/CD44v6 interactions and reduction in adenoma growth in Apc Min/+ MICE. J Biolog Chem 2009; 284(18): 12432-46. [PMID: 19246453]

[101] Askarian S, Abnous K, Taghavi S, Oskuee RK, Ramezani M. Cellular delivery of shRNA using aptamer-conjugated PLL-alkyl-PEI nanoparticles. Colloids and Surfaces B: Biointerfaces 2015; 136: 355-64.

[102] Chu TC, Twu KY, Ellington AD, Levy M. Aptamer mediated siRNA delivery. Nucl Acids Res 2006; 34(10): e73-e. [http://dx.doi.org/10.1093/nar/gkl388]

[103] Dassie JP, Liu X-y, Thomas GS, Whitaker RM, Thiel KW, Stockdale KR, *et al.* ystemic administration of optimized aptamer-siRNA chimeras promotes regression of PSMA-expressing tumors. Nature Biotechn 2009; 27(9): 839-46.

[104] Behlke MA. Chemical modification of siRNAs for in vivo use. Oligonucleotides 2008; 18(4): 305-19. [http://dx.doi.org/10.1089/oli.2008.0164] [PMID: 19025401]

[105] Soundararajan S, Chen W, Spicer EK, Courtenay-Luck N, Fernandes DJ. The nucleolin targeting aptamer AS1411 destabilizes Bcl-2 messenger RNA in human breast cancer cells. Cancer Res 2008; 68(7): 2358-65. [http://dx.doi.org/10.1158/0008-5472.CAN-07-5723] [PMID: 18381443]

[106] Reynolds A, Leake D, Boese Q, Scaringe S, Marshall WS, Khvorova A. Rational siRNA design for RNA interference. Nature Biotechn 2004; 22(3): 326-30. [http://dx.doi.org/10.1038/nbt936]

[107] Niu S, Zhang L-K, Zhang L, Zhuang S, Zhan X, Chen W-Y, *et al.* Inhibition by multifunctional magnetic nanoparticles loaded with alpha-synuclein RNAi plasmid in a parkinson. Theranostics 2017; 7(2):344.

[108] Wu Y, Yu J, Liu Y, *et al.* Delivery of EZH2-shRNA with mPEG-PEI nanoparticles for the treatment of prostate cancer *in vitro*. Int J Mol Med 2014; 33(6): 1563-9. [http://dx.doi.org/10.3892/ijmm.2014.1724] [PMID: 24714818]

[109] Yang AQ, Wang PJ, Huang T, Zhou WL, Landman J. Effects of monomethoxypolyethylene glycol-chitosan nanoparticle-mediated dual silencing of livin and survivin genes in prostate cancer PC-3M cells. Genetics and Mol Res: GMR 2016; 15(2).

[PMID: 27173182]

[110] Zhang MX, Hong SS, Cai QQ, *et al.* Transcriptional control of the MUC16 promoter facilitates follicle-stimulating hormone peptide-conjugated shRNA nanoparticle-mediated inhibition of ovarian carcinoma *in vivo*. Drug Deliv 2018; 25(1): 797-806. [http://dx.doi.org/10.1080/10717544.2018.1451934] [PMID: 29542355]

[111] Hong SS, Zhang MX, Zhang M, *et al.* Follicle-stimulating hormone peptide-conjugated nanoparticles for targeted shRNA delivery lead to effective gro-α silencing and antitumor activity against ovarian cancer. Drug Deliv 2018; 25(1): 576-84. [http://dx.doi.org/10.1080/10717544.2018.1440667] [PMID: 29461120]

[112] Ayatollahi S, Salmasi Z, Hashemi M, Askarian S, Oskuee RK, Abnous K, *et al.* Aptamer-targeted delivery of Bcl-xL shRNA using alkyl modified PAMAM dendrimers into lung cancer cells. Int J biochem Cell bio 2017; 92: 210-7. [http://dx.doi.org/10.1016/j.biocel.2017.10.005]

[113] Li Z, Zhang L, Tang C, Yin C. Co-delivery of doxorubicin and survivin shRNA-expressing plasmid *via* microenvironment-responsive dendritic mesoporous silica nanoparticles for synergistic cancer therapy. Pharmaceut Res 2017; 34(12): 2829-41. [http://dx.doi.org/10.1007/s11095-017-2264-6]

[114] Hu Q, Li W, Hu X, Hu Q, Shen J, Jin X, *et al.* Synergistic treatment of ovarian cancer by co-delivery of survivin shRNA and paclitaxel via supramolecular micellar assembly. Biomat 2012; 33(27): 6580-91. [http://dx.doi.org/10.1016/j.biomaterials.2012.05.060]

[115] Taghavi S, HashemNia A, Mosaffa F, *et al.* Preparation and evaluation of polyethylenimine-functionalized carbon nanotubes tagged with 5TR1 aptamer for targeted delivery of Bcl-xL shRNA into breast cancer cells. Colloids and Surfaces B: Biointerfaces 2016; 140: 28-39.

[116] Yin Q, Gao Y, Zhang Z, Zhang P, Li Y. Bioreducible poly (β-amino esters)/shRNA complex nanoparticles for efficient RNA delivery. J Control Rel 2011; 151(1): 35-44.

[117] Yang Y, Gao Y, Chen L, Huang Y, Li Y. Downregulation of survivin expression and enhanced chemosensitivity of MCF-7 cells to adriamycin by PDMAE/survivin shRNA complex nanoparticles. Intern J Pharmaceu 2011; 405(1): 188-95.

[118] Jere D, Xu C X, Arote R, Yun C H, Cho M H, Cho C S. Poly(β amino ester) as a carrier for si/shRNA delivery in lung cancer cells. Biomater 2008; 29(16): 2535-47.

[119] Taghavi S, Nia AH, Abnous K, Ramezani M. Polyethylenimine-functionalized carbon nanotubes tagged with AS1411 aptamer for combination gene and drug delivery into human gastric cancer cells. Intern J Pharmaceu 2017; 516(1): 301-12. [http://dx.doi.org/10.1016/j.ijpharm.2016.11.027]

[120] Singh S, Narang AS, Mahato RI. Subcellular Fate and Off-Target Effects of siRNA, shRNA, and miRNA. Pharmaceutical Res 2011; 28(12): 2996-3015. [http://dx.doi.org/10.1007/s11095-011-0608-1]

[121] Lares MR, Rossi JJ, Ouellet DL. RNAi and small interfering RNAs in human disease therapeutic applications. Trends Biotechnol 2010; 28(11): 570-9. [http://dx.doi.org/10.1016/j.tibtech.2010.07.009] [PMID: 20833440]

[122] Maples P, Kumar P, Yu Y, Wang Z, Jay C, Pappen B, *et al.* FANG vaccine: autologous tumor cell vaccine genetically modified to express GM-CSF and block production of furin. BioProcessing J 2010; 8: 4-14.

[123] van Es JH, Barker N, Clevers H. You Wnt some, you lose some: oncogenes in the Wnt signaling pathway. Curr Opin Genet Dev 2003; 13(1): 28-33. [http://dx.doi.org/10.1016/S0959-437X(02)00012-6]

CHAPTER 8

miRNA and Nanoparticle Conjugate as a Future Therapeutic Approach

Abstract: Micro RNAs are naturally occurring RNA molecules that help in the degradation of mRNA molecules sequence specifically. They degrade the mRNA molecules and thus inhibit the formation of protein after translation. miRNA expression varies from tissue to tissue and from one disease condition to other. Thus this molecule becomes a target of therapy in various types of disease conditions. But, the use of bare miRNAs has several drawbacks as they may degrade in the body fluid due to their fragile nature. So, in this regard nanoparticles have a very vital role to overcome these disadvantages. In this study, we intended to discuss the various forms of miRNA therapeutic approaches, along with various types of nanoparticles that may carry the miRNA and its antagomirs to the target site.

Keywords: Aptamer nanoparticle, Chitosan nanoparticle, Circulating miRNA, Cyclodextrin nanoparticle, Dendrimer nanoparticle, Gold nanoparticle, Graphine nanoparticle, Inorganic nanoparticle, Lipid nanoparticle, miRNA, miRNA replacement therapy, miRNA suppression therapy, Magnetic nanoparticle, Mesoporous silica nanoparticle, Off target effect, Organic nanoparticle, PLGA nanoparticle, Polyethyleneimine nanoparticle, Polymeric nanoparticle, Protein nanoparticle, Quantum dote nanoparticle, Stability.

INTRODUCTION

Micro RNAs are 18-25 nucleotide sequence that binds at the 3' untranslated region of the mRNA molecule that makes them double stranded and ultimately degrades them [1, 2]. miRNAs participate in several functions of the body that includes development, viral defense, organogenesis, cell proliferation/apoptosis, hematopoietic processes and fat metabolism [3 - 6]. Lee *et al.*, first time in 1993 identified miRNA in *C. elegans via* genetic screening [7]. Since then, a wide variety of miRNAs have been identified in a large number of organisms.

miRNAs originating from tissue can exist in various parts of the body. They may exist in tissues or in the circulating body fluids.

Rituparna Acharya

Tissue Specific Expression

miRNAs may be expressed in tissues of various organs [8]. Specific tissues have specific expression pattern of miRNAs. Even in tumor tissues, the miRNA expression is of aberrant type. Depending upon the expression profile of the miRNAs, tumor tissues are diagnosed, graded and the prognosis of the tumor is made [9]. Even in many higher plants and animals, this miRNA is found to be expressed widely and varies from one tissue to the other [10].

Circulation miRNAs

Current research has revealed that miRNAs not only exist in the tissues but also in various body fluids [11]. By using expression profiling of these miRNAs in the body, fluid various forms of diseases are diagnosed that identify specific biomarkers for specific disease conditions [12]. Recent evidences have indicated that these circulating miRNAs within microvesicles may enter within the cell and affect the expression level of the target gene (Fig. **1**) [13].

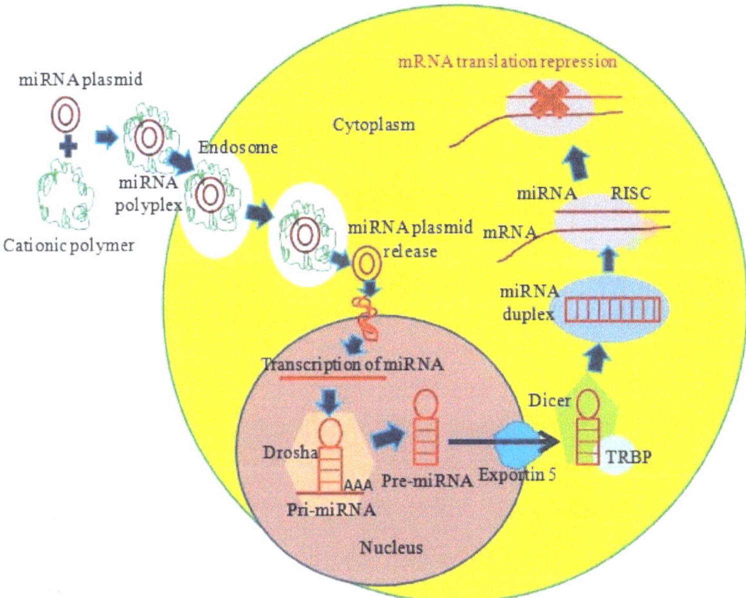

Fig. (1). Mechanism of action of miRNA plasmid-nanoparticle conjugate.

In our study, we will discuss the use of miRNAs for therapeutic purposes. Different therapeutic approaches are discussed in the next section of the study.

THERAPEUTIC APPROACHES USING MIRNAS

Bare RNAs are highly susceptible to degradation in the blood by enzymes and may get phagocytized by many phagocytic cells. Using nanoparticles may increase the stability of the RNAs *in vivo*. Antisense oligonucleotide technology is nothing but the study of miRNAs and technology that silences the miRNAs is known as anti-miRNA oligonucleotide technology [14].

To change the expression of the target gene, the miRNA therapies may be of two types-one is the miRNA suppression therapy and the second is the miRNA replacement therapy.

miRNA Suppression Therapy

Through this therapy, the suppression of the mRNA by miRNAs is removed that increases the expression level of the mRNAs. Anti-miRNA oligonucleotide binds with the sense strand of the miRNA and resists their interaction with the miRISC complex. Thus the complexes are blocked to interact with the mRNAs and prevent their degradation, so, the mRNA expression is upregulated. To increase the stability and affinity of the antagomirs and miRNA inhibitors, nanoparticles may be used.

miRNA inhibitors also known as anti-miRNAs are single stranded RNA molecules that bindwith the endogenous miRNAs and abolish their activities on mRNAs. miRNA inhibitors are usually used *in vitro* in combination with lipofectamines that makes them internalize by the cells.

Antagomirs are the RNA molecules with certain chemical modifications that make them stable and cellular uptake is easy [15]. This may be used *in vivo* in local and systemic administration to down regulate the specific miRNA expression.

miRNA masks are a special type of single stranded ribonucleic acid that have 2′-O-methyl-modifications [16]. This RNA molecule does not bind directly with the miRNA but to the 3’-UTR of the target mRNA molecule. miRNA masks are suitable for research applications.

miRNA sponges are the special type of plasmid encoding RNAs that have the complementary sequence of the seed region of the miRNAs [17]. After the transfection within the cells, this plasmid transcribes sponge RNAs that binds with the miRNAs that have same seed sequence. Thus the miRNA expression is inhibited and the subsequent mRNA expression is upregulated as a result.

miRNA Replacement Therapy

miRNA mimics are the double-stranded miRNA like RNA molecules that binds with the target mRNA molecules and modify the post transcriptional mRNAs.

miRNAagomirs are double-stranded miRNA mimics that have certain chemical modifications as antagomirs. These chemical modifications help in the stability and affinity of the miRNA molecules that upregulate the miRNAs *in vivo*.

Another method of upregulating miRNAs is by the help of miRNA precursors. These single stranded precursors are transfected within the cell by lipofectamin or electroporation that leads to the cleavage of the precursor by dicer enzyme and formation of mature miRNAs.

miRNA expressing plasmids are another method of replacement therapy. The plasmids may carry fluorescent reporter gene that helps in the localization of the miRNA molecules.

The chemical modification of these miRNAs may increase their stability and affinity but that is not sufficient for *in vivo* applications (Fig. **2**).

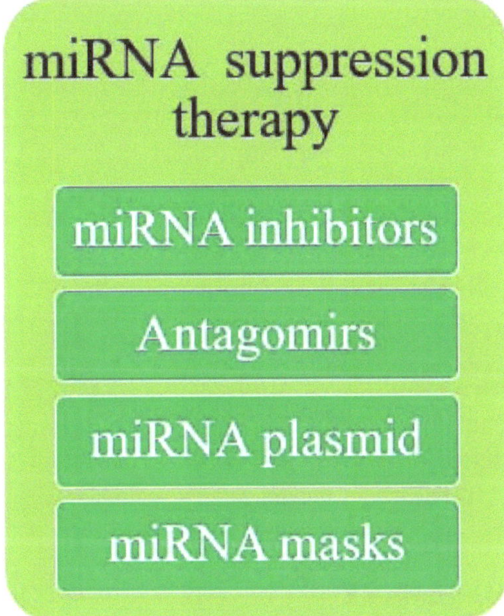

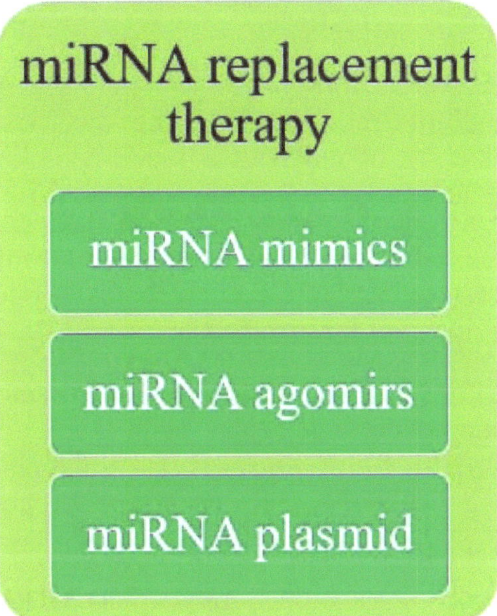

Fig. (2). Therapeutic approaches using miRNA.

CHALLENGES IN MIRNA BASED THERAPIES

The advancement of RNA innovation has started considering miRNA as a new therapeutic molecule. Repressing gene expression is the main attribute of the miRNA molecules that may be used for a pharmacological application research. But while using these RNA molecules *in vivo* leads to many challenges and hurdles on its way of optimum use. We are intended to discuss all the challenges that are faced by the researchers while using them in a bare form.

Instability within Blood Vascular System

The main challenge of using miRNAs and its other bare forms is rapid degradation of these molecules in the blood. For therapeutic applications, if these bare molecules are administered systemically, they have a very short half-life and they degrade rapidly in contact with the widespread nucleases present in the blood and vascular system.

Reduced Intracellular Delivery

Another hurdle of using bare miRNA and its forms is their inability to be permeable within the cell. As these molecules pose high molecular weight and negative charges, they are impermeable to the cell membrane.

Off Target Effects

As single miRNA targets multiple genes and a single gene is regulated by multiple miRNAs [18], the specificity of the miRNAs is very low. So, the function of miRNAs is much complicated than what was supposed to be.

To overcome these challenges, nanoparticles play a vital role. They can increase the stability and half-life of the molecules. At the same time, they can increase the permeability of these molecules through cell membrane and help in the targeted delivery of these molecules.

In this study, we will discuss the nanoparticles and their application in miRNA suppression and replacement therapy. These nanoparticles may be divided into several forms such as (1) inorganic material-based delivery systems, (2) organic/lipid-based nanocarriers, (3) polymeric vectors/dendrimer based vectors.

NANOPARTICLE ASSISTED MIRNA DELIVERY

Recent years the advancement of nanotechnology developed many novel materials and applied them in multiple numbers of novel sites [19]. These progresses in research have developed many DNA, RNA delivery vehicles for the treatment of several disease conditions. These wide varieties of inorganic, organic and polymeric nanomaterials are developing as a vector for the delivery of these macromolecules. These nanomaterial vectors have several advantages such as they may be nontoxic and biocompatible, they are non-immunogenic and flexible in their design depending upon the target site [20].

Inorganic Nanoparticle Based Delivery of miRNA and Anti-miRNA

Inorganic nanoparticles may be made tailor make depending upon their site of delivery. They are made highly nontoxic and biocompatible with biodegradable properties. Their size, shape and surface properties may be altered depending upon the macromolecule they will carry. They have unique electrical and optical properties as well [21].

Gold Nanoconjugate

Gold nanoparticles have high potential for the application in the therapeutic field due to their unique properties such as they are easy to synthesis, inactive in nature, highly functionalized, high absorption coefficient and ability to target a tissue. Therefore they have a wide variety of potential application in the field of medicine and gene delivery. Due to their remarkable ability to be stable in the blood, possessing large surface area, formulating surface structure and biocompatibility make them as able nanoparticle for gene delivery. The anionic nature of the bare miRNAs produces a challenge in the delivery of them through the cell membrane and reduces the half-life of them in the blood vascular system. To make them permeable through the cell membrane lipofectamine and electroporation is needed. To address these challenges gold nanoparticle demonstrate a vital role as they show nontoxic property to the cell, they demonstrate to carry large payloads and show faster endosomal escape and longer half-life [22].

Graphine Nanoconjugate

Graphine nanoparticles have unique optical, thermal and electrical properties [23]. They are found to be highly efficient chemotherapeutic drug delivery vehicle and gene targeting agent for example the targeting of miRNAs to cancer cells [24].

Mesoporous Silica Nanoconjugate

Silica is also used as a delivery vehicle for miRNAs. Mesoporous silica has large pore size and surface area that makes them an ideal gene delivery vehicle [25]. miR-122 antagomir and miR-34a was delivered through this nanoparticle demonstrated to be delivered to the target tissue [26]. Li *et.al.,* demonstrated the delivery of anti-miRNA-155 loaded mesoporous silica nanoparticle with others as an effective suppressor of colorectal cancer in mouse model [27].

Quantum Dot Nanoconjugate

Quantum dotes are nanocrystals with monodispers and semiconductor property [28] that may be synthesized by colloidal and plasma synthesis method [29]. miR-26a as a payload it demonstrated arrest of cell cycle and inhibition of cancer cell proliferation [30]. It showed that quantum dotes may be used as a miRNA delivery method for the treatment of cancer and other types of disease conditions.

Magnetic Nanoconjugate

Magnetic nanoparticle Fe3O4 was developed for the delivery of miRNA-100 in conjugation with polymers (poly (γ-glutamicacid) (γ-PGA), polyacrylic acid (PAA) or polyethylenimine (PEI)). Due to the mesoporous structure of this polymer made them deal for gene delivery and miRNA loading as well as rapid tumor cell uptake. Moreover in addition with the delivery of chemotherapeutic drugs made them potent anticancer agent [31].

Organic Nanoparticle Based Delivery of miRNA and Anti-miRNA

Organic nanoparticles are mainly derived from animal and vegetable sources [32 - 34]. They are mainly made up of carbon and are highly biocompatible, non-cytotoxic and non-immunogenic [35, 36]. They rapidly interact with oppositely charged molecules such as siRNAs and miRNAs with high loading capacity of the payload [37].

Chitosan Based Nanoconjugate

Chitosan is generated from the deacetylation of the chitin from crustacean shell. It is highly used as miRNA delivery vehicle due to its biocompatibility, cationic nature and abundance in environment [38, 39]. Publications demonstrated chitosan as a delivery vehicle of miR-34a and doxorubicin for the treatment of breast cancer [40]. Also miRNA-124 delivery through chitosan decreased the abundance of microglial cells in spinal injury in rats [41].

Lipid/liposome Based Nanoconjugate

Lipids may be easily modified to make them conjugate with variety of nucleotides for delivering them *in vivo*. Cationic lipids are the main delivery vehicle for DNA/RNA/miRNAs to the endoplasmic reticular system of the human being [42, 43]. They are easy to handle, non-toxic and produces less immunogenic reactions as a non-viral delivery media [44, 45]. However, these cationic lipid nanoparticles have low delivery efficiency that is the main obstacle for their clinical application. To overcome this drawback new formulations have developed using lipid nanoparticles. Modified lipid nanoparticles are used in conjugation with anti-mi--155 to hepatocellular carcinoma [46]. Cationic lipid nanoparticles are also used in conjugation with miR-122 mimic to upregulate that miRNA in hepatocellular carcinoma [45]. Lipid based nanoparticles are also used to deliver mimic miR-34a or miR 143/145 in pancreatic cancer [47]. miR29b or miR 133b was also used for the treatment of lung cancer [48]. Pre-miR-107 was used to inhibit head and neck squamous cell carcinoma [49]. Lipid based nanoparticle was also used to prevent neovascularization by the help of anti-miR-296 [50]. Tokyo university researchers demonstrated the use of miRNA-126 loaded in modified liposomal nanoparticle in promoting angiogenesis in ischemic model [51]. In a murine breast cancer model miR-10b antagomir demonstrated reduced tumor growth and delayed lung metastasis [52].

Protein or Peptide Based Nanoconjugate

As a nucleic acid delivery vehicle proteins and peptides are widely explored. The positively charged amino acids have an electrostatic interaction with the negatively charged RNA molecules. Further they have an added facility for the endosomal escape and targeted delivery [53]. Peptide mediated delivery of anti-miR-21 in gliobastoma in an animal model was studied [54, 55]. Anti-cancer effect of miR-29b was also studied by Suh *et.al* [56]. Peptide based nanoconjugate with anti-miR-199a was used to inhibit pancreatic cancer [57].

Aptamers Nanoconjugate

Aptamers are three dimensional DNA or RNA molecules that may be targeted to macromolecules, specific tissue, organelle or even organism with high affinity [58]. Aptamers have high specificity with wide variety of target molecules. Moreover they are highly stable in blood and produce less immunogenic reaction. miR-29b was used in conjugation with the aptamer in ovarian cancer [59]. Anti-miR-17 was used to treat prostate cancer in conjugation with aptamer [60]. Anti-miR-21 was used in breast cancer [61]. miR-212 down regulated several genes in lung cancer [62]. miR-26a protected tumor growth in absence of chemotherapy [63].

Polymeric Nanoparticle Based Delivery of miRNA and Anti-miRNA

Natural and synthetic polymers have variation in their physiochemical properties. Wide variety of polymers has taken attention for the delivery of payload to the target organ. Polymeric nanoparticles have several advantages over the other organic nanoparticles such as they are highly stable in the body fluid. Moreover they are highly suitable for industrial scale up as they have short preparation time. The synthetic polymers include dendrimers, polyphosphoesters and polyethyleneimines.

Polyethyleneimine Nanoconjugate

This nanoparticle is the most studied material for gene delivery as they have their unique property of buffering limit [64]. They may be linear or brunched in their structure. Few studies have demonstrated the delivery of miRNAs through this nanoparticle [65 - 67]. Significant anti-tumor effect was found in the colon carcinoma mouse xenograft model when miR-145 and miR-33a mimic was administered in conjugation with Polyethyleneimine [68]. Moreover, miR-141 and miR-31 precursors demonstrated increased level of these miRNAs in colon tissue when administered through intracolonic route [69, 70].

Dendrimer Nanoconjugate

Dendrimers are highly branched macromolecules that have nano size and mono disperse characteristics. They are a vitally important polymer that helps in the delivery of genetic materials [71]. They may encapsulate or conjugate with the payload and deliver it to the target organ. PAMAM dendrimer was used to deliver miR-7 to brain glioma cells demonstrated high transfection efficiency and improved therapeutic application *in vitro* and *in vivo* [72]. Moreover, codelivery of anti-miR- 21 and 5'-fluorouracil showed reduced cytotoxicity and migration, further improved the apoptosis of glioblastoma cells [73]. When miR-126 was delivered it reduced the proliferation of the cells [74]. Further through intravenous injection of miR-21 in conjugation with dendrimers showed high level of efficacy [75].

PLGA Based Nanoconjugate

PLGA nanoparticles have several characteristics such as they are water insoluble, they have high loading capacity [76] and they protect the nucleic acids from degradation [77]. Moreover, they are safe biodegradable and have the history of their use as a therapeutic agent [78]. Anti-miR-10b and anti-miR-21 acts as an anti-tumor agent in mice model [79]. Co-delivery of anti-miR-21 and gemcitabine demonstrated therapeutic efficacy in hepatocellular carcinoma [79]. Moreover, co-delivery of doxorubicin and miR-542-3p showed efficacy in breast cancer [80].

Further, in breast cancer the combined delivery of orlistat loaded nanoparticles and anti-miR-21 or doxorubicin loaded nanoparticles demonstrated apoptosis [81]. In neurodegenerative disease also miR-124-PLGA nanoconjugate showed gainful insights [82].

Cyclodextrin Nanoconjugate

Cyclodextrin is a carbohydrate based nanoparticle that has high efficiency in delivering miRNAs [83]. A novel delivery vehicle was composed by Zeng *et al.* by using matrixmetalloproteinase-2 (MMP2)-cleavable substrate peptides in conjugate with miRNA-34a mimics. This conjugate has excellent tumor targeting and anti-tumor activity [84].

CHALLENGES WITH RNA NANOTECHNOLOGY

Construction of nanoparticle in conjugation with RNA molecules needs many chemical modifications. Although we have become successful in producing nanoconjugates comprising of nanoparticle and RNA molecule there are more scope of improvement in this field. There are many hurdles that need to overcome in the area of nanotechnology that comprises of RNA-nanoparticle conjugate.

Challenge in RNA Structure Prediction

The major area of challenge in the field of RNA nanotechnology is the prediction of accurate 3-D structure of the RNA-nanoparticle conjugate. The 2-D structure prediction program predicts only 70% of the original structure [85, 86]. The actual folding pattern of the RNA molecule within the nanoparticle is still under research. Bioinformatics tools with the help of many software programs are trying to predict the structure but more refinement is needed [87 - 89].

Stability of the Nanoconjugate

RNA molecules are highly susceptible to nuclease (RNases) activity in the blood vascular system. In this regards, to make this molecules stable several formulations of nanoparticles have been developed. When these RNA molecules are intercalated within the nanoparticles they become stable in the blood. Moreover, along with this strategy several other chemical modifications have been tried to make them stable in the harsh environment [90 - 92].

In Vivo Half-life and Retention Time of the Nanoconjugate

It has been suggested that 10-100nm of size is optimum for non-viral delivery of RNAs. Although this range is large enough to retain within the body and small enough to bind with the cellular receptors and for cellular uptake. So, optimum size of the RNA-nanoparticle conjugate is important for half-life and retention within the body [93]. The half-life is found to be optimized at 5-10h but there are more scope of improvement [94].

Limited Carrying Capacity of the Nanoparticle

Presently, limited carrying capacities of the nanoparticles are a major limitation on the delivery of large molecular weight RNA molecules. Recently, many nanoparticles have been fabricated to carry larger payloads to the target organ. However, the nanoparticles with low carrying capacity are usually non-toxic [95]. So, nanoparticles with large carrying capacity but making them non-toxic all together are a major challenge of today's research.

Scaling Up of the Conjugate

Expensive production cost of RNA-nanoparticle conjugate has reduced their application in medicine. Although, the production of oligonucleotides have reduced due to the advancement of the technology; but large scale purification still remains as a problem. Gel electrophoresis and liquid chromatography are effective in low yield cases. Recently ultracentrifugation is being employed for high yield of RNA-nanoparticle conjugate [96].

Hurdles in Endosomal Escape of the Payload

Receptor mediated endocytosis is one of the well-established way of RNA delivery within the cell. However in cancer therapy it has been [97] found that the escape of RNA from RNA-nanoparticle conjugate is still a problem [98]. Various methods have been employed but more need to be done as the need of the hour [99].

CONCLUSION

A wide variety of nanoparticles as a delivery vehicle of RNA have been developed recently. The main attribute of these nanoparticles is to deliver the RNA molecules to the target organ without being affected by nucleases in the serum and without producing adverse immune responses. Most of the studies have used the intravenous and local route of administration and few of them have used oral route. Fabrication of the nanoparticle to optimize the stability and cellular uptake of the RNAs was used. The main challenge of systemic administration is when these cargos are administered, they are readily captured by liver and spleen and are eliminated by kidney. To increase the efficiency of delivery may only be achieved by increasing the longevity of the nanoconjugate in the blood and making them efficient in targeting the site of specificity. Therefore, to optimize these aspects of delivery, new biomaterials should be developed. The ideal biomaterial is liposomal delivery that has higher biocompatibility and negligible immunogenicity. To materialize and optimize this delivery vehicle, the all over understanding of the biological system is of utmost importance .

REFERENCES

[1] Bartel DP. MicroRNAs: genomics, biogenesis, mechanism, and function. Cell 2004; 116(2): 281-97. [http://dx.doi.org/10.1016/S0092-8674(04)00045-5] [PMID: 14744438]

[2] He L, Hannon GJ. MicroRNAs: small RNAs with a big role in gene regulation. Nat Rev Genet 2004; 5(7): 522-31. [http://dx.doi.org/10.1038/nrg1379] [PMID: 15211354]

[3] O'Connell RM, Rao DS, Chaudhuri AA, Baltimore D. Physiological and pathological roles for microRNAs in the immune system. Nat Rev Immunol 2010; 10(2): 111-22. [http://dx.doi.org/10.1038/nri2708] [PMID: 20098459]

[4] Lu J, Getz G, Miska EA, *et al.* MicroRNA expression profiles classify human cancers. Nature 2005; 435(7043): 834-8. [http://dx.doi.org/10.1038/nature03702] [PMID: 15944708]

[5] Jeang KT. RNAi in the regulation of mammalian viral infections. BMC Biol 2012; 10: 58. [http://dx.doi.org/10.1186/1741-7007-10-58] [PMID: 22734679]

[6] Rottiers V, Näär AM. MicroRNAs in metabolism and metabolic disorders. Nat Rev Mol Cell Biol 2012; 13(4): 239-50. [http://dx.doi.org/10.1038/nrm3313] [PMID: 22436747]

[7] Lee RC, Feinbaum RL, Ambros V. The C. elegans heterochronic gene lin-4 encodes small RNAs with antisense complementarity to lin-14. Cell 1993; 75(5): 843-54. [http://dx.doi.org/10.1016/0092-8674(93)90529-Y] [PMID: 8252621]

[8] Wienholds E, Kloosterman WP, Miska E, *et al.* MicroRNA expression in zebrafish embryonic development. Science 2005; 309(5732): 310-1. [http://dx.doi.org/10.1126/science.1114519] [PMID: 15919954]

[9] Cheng WT, Rosario R, Muthukaruppan A, *et al.* MicroRNA profiling of ovarian granulosa cell tumours reveals novel diagnostic and prognostic markers. Clin Epigenetics 2017; 9: 72. [http://dx.doi.org/10.1186/s13148-017-0372-0] [PMID: 28736583]

[10] Xu L, Hu Y, Cao Y, *et al.* An expression atlas of miRNAs in Arabidopsis thaliana. Sci China Life Sci 2018; 61(2): 178-89. [http://dx.doi.org/10.1007/s11427-017-9199-1] [PMID: 29197026]

[11] Lawrie CH, Gal S, Dunlop HM, *et al.* Detection of elevated levels of tumour-associated microRNAs in serum of patients with diffuse large B-cell lymphoma. Br J Haematol 2008; 141(5): 672-5. [http://dx.doi.org/10.1111/j.1365-2141.2008.07077.x] [PMID: 18318758]

[12] Chen X, Ba Y, Ma L, *et al.* Characterization of microRNAs in serum: a novel class of biomarkers for diagnosis of cancer and other diseases. Cell Res 2008; 18(10): 997-1006. [http://dx.doi.org/10.1038/cr.2008.282] [PMID: 18766170]

[13] Jung HJ, Suh Y. Circulating miRNAs in ageing and ageing-related diseases. J Genet Genomics 2014; 41(9): 465-72. [PMID: 25269672]

[14] Zhang B, Farwell MA. microRNAs: a new emerging class of players for disease diagnostics and gene therapy. J Cell Mol Med 2008; 12(1): 3-21. [http://dx.doi.org/10.1111/j.1582-4934.2007.00196.x] [PMID: 18088390]

[15] Krützfeldt J, Rajewsky N, Braich R, Rajeev K, Tuschl T, Manoharan M, *et al.* Silencing of microRNAs in vivo with 'antagomirs'. Nature 2006; 438: 685-9.

[16] Wang Z. The principles of MiRNA-masking antisense oligonucleotides technology. Methods Mol Biol 2011; 676: 43-9.
[http://dx.doi.org/10.1007/978-1-60761-863-8_3] [PMID: 20931388]

[17] Kluiver J, Slezak-Prochazka I, Smigielska-Czepiel K, Halsema N, Kroesen BJ, van den Berg A. Generation of miRNA sponge constructs. Methods 2012; 58(2): 113-7.
[http://dx.doi.org/10.1016/j.ymeth.2012.07.019] [PMID: 22836127]

[18] Guo P, Haque F, Hallahan B, Reif R, Li H. Uniqueness, advantages, challenges, solutions, and perspectives in therapeutics applying RNA nanotechnology. Nucleic Acid Ther 2012; 22(4): 226-45.
[http://dx.doi.org/10.1089/nat.2012.0350] [PMID: 22913595]

[19] Biju V. Chemical modifications and bioconjugate reactions of nanomaterials for sensing, imaging, drug delivery and therapy. Chem Soc Rev 2014; 43(3): 744-64.
[http://dx.doi.org/10.1039/C3CS60273G] [PMID: 24220322]

[20] Riley MK, Vermerris W. Recent advances in nanomaterials for gene delivery-a review. Nanomaterials (Basel) 2017; 7(5): 94.
[http://dx.doi.org/10.3390/nano7050094] [PMID: 28452950]

[21] Prasad P, Masters B. Introduction to biophotonics. J Biomed Optics 2005; 10: 39901.
[http://dx.doi.org/10.1117/1.1931672]

[22] Ghosh R, Singh LC, Shohet JM, Gunaratne PH. A gold nanoparticle platform for the delivery of functional microRNAs into cancer cells. Biomaterials 2013; 34(3): 807-16.
[http://dx.doi.org/10.1016/j.biomaterials.2012.10.023] [PMID: 23111335]

[23] Lu CH, Yang HH, Zhu CL, Chen X, Chen GN. A graphene platform for sensing biomolecules. Angew Chem Int Ed Engl 2009; 48(26): 4785-7.
[http://dx.doi.org/10.1002/anie.200901479] [PMID: 19475600]

[24] Yang HW, Huang CY, Lin CW, *et al.* Gadolinium-functionalized nanographene oxide for combined drug and microRNA delivery and magnetic resonance imaging. Biomaterials 2014; 35(24): 6534-42.
[http://dx.doi.org/10.1016/j.biomaterials.2014.04.057] [PMID: 24811259]

[25] Wang Z, Wu P, He Z, *et al.* Mesoporous silica nanoparticles with lactose-mediated targeting effect to deliver platinum(iv) prodrug for liver cancer therapy. J Mater Chem B Mater Biol Med 2017; 5(36): 7591-7.
[http://dx.doi.org/10.1039/C7TB01704A] [PMID: 32264234]

[26] Tivnan A, Orr WS, Gubala V, *et al.* Inhibition of neuroblastoma tumor growth by targeted delivery of microRNA-34a using anti-disialoganglioside GD2 coated nanoparticles. PLoS One 2012; 7(5): e38129.
[http://dx.doi.org/10.1371/journal.pone.0038129] [PMID: 22662276]

[27] Li Y, Duo Y, Bi J, *et al.* Targeted delivery of anti-miR-155 by functionalized mesoporous silica nanoparticles for colorectal cancer therapy. Int J Nanomedicine 2018; 13: 1241-56.
[http://dx.doi.org/10.2147/IJN.S158290] [PMID: 29535520]

[28] Murray CB, Norris DJ, Bawendi MG. Synthesis and characterization of nearly monodisperse CdE (E = sulfur, selenium, tellurium) semiconductor nanocrystallites. J Americ Chemical Soc 1993; 115(19): 8706-15.

[29] Kortshagen U. Nonthermal plasma synthesis of semiconductor nanocrystals. J Physics D: Applied Physics 2009; 42: 113001.
[http://dx.doi.org/10.1088/0022-3727/42/11/113001]

[30] Liang G, Li Y, Feng W, *et al.* Polyethyleneimine-coated quantum dots for miRNA delivery and its enhanced suppression in HepG2 cells. Int J Nanomedicine 2016; 11: 6079-88.

[http://dx.doi.org/10.2147/IJN.S120828] [PMID: 27895481]

[31] Sun S, Wang Y, Zhou R, *et al.* Targeting and Regulating of an Oncogene via Nanovector Delivery of MicroRNA using Patient-Derived Xenografts. Theranostics 2017; 7(3): 677-93. [http://dx.doi.org/10.7150/thno.16357] [PMID: 28255359]

[32] Prabaharan M, Mano JF. Chitosan-based particles as controlled drug delivery systems. Drug Deliv 2005; 12(1): 41-57. [http://dx.doi.org/10.1080/10717540590889781] [PMID: 15801720]

[33] Hu L, Sun Y, Wu Y. Advances in chitosan-based drug delivery vehicles. Nanoscale 2013; 5(8): 3103-11. [http://dx.doi.org/10.1039/c3nr00338h] [PMID: 23515527]

[34] Bernkop-Schnürch A, Dünnhaupt S. Chitosan-based drug delivery systems. Europ J Pharmaceu and Biopharmaceu 2012; 81(3): 463-9. [http://dx.doi.org/10.1016/j.ejpb.2012.04.007]

[35] Costa DF, Torchilin VP. Micelle-like nanoparticles as siRNA and miRNA carriers for cancer therapy. Biomed Microdevices 2018; 20(3): 59. [http://dx.doi.org/10.1007/s10544-018-0298-0] [PMID: 29998417]

[36] Bravo-Anaya LM, Fernández-Solís KG, Rosselgong J, Nano-Rodríguez JLE, Carvajal F, Rinaudo M. Chitosan-DNA polyelectrolyte complex: Influence of chitosan characteristics and mechanism of complex formation. Int J Biol Macromol 2019; 126: 1037-49. [http://dx.doi.org/10.1016/j.ijbiomac.2019.01.008] [PMID: 30615969]

[37] Layek B, Lipp L, Singh J. Cell penetrating peptide conjugated chitosan for enhanced delivery of nucleic acid. Int J Mol Sci 2015; 16(12): 28912-30. [http://dx.doi.org/10.3390/ijms161226142] [PMID: 26690119]

[38] Mao S, Sun W, Kissel T. Chitosan-based formulations for delivery of DNA and siRNA. Adv Drug Deliv Rev 2010; 62(1): 12-27. [http://dx.doi.org/10.1016/j.addr.2009.08.004] [PMID: 19796660]

[39] Garcia-Fuentes M, Alonso MJ. Chitosan-based drug nanocarriers: where do we stand? J. Control. Release Soc 2012; 161(2): 496-504. [http://dx.doi.org/10.1016/j.jconrel.2012.03.017] [PMID: 22480607]

[40] Deng X, Cao M, Zhang J, *et al.* Hyaluronic acid-chitosan nanoparticles for co-delivery of MiR-34a and doxorubicin in therapy against triple negative breast cancer. Biomaterials 2014; 35(14): 4333-44. [http://dx.doi.org/10.1016/j.biomaterials.2014.02.006] [PMID: 24565525]

[41] Louw AM, Kolar MK, Novikova LN, *et al.* Chitosan polyplex mediated delivery of miRNA-124 reduces activation of microglial cells *in vitro* and in rat models of spinal cord injury. Nanomedicine (Lond) 2016; 12(3): 643-53. [http://dx.doi.org/10.1016/j.nano.2015.10.011] [PMID: 26582736]

[42] Ewert K, Slack NL, Ahmad A, *et al.* Cationic lipid-DNA complexes for gene therapy: understanding the relationship between complex structure and gene delivery pathways at the molecular level. Curr Med Chem 2004; 11(2): 133-49. [http://dx.doi.org/10.2174/0929867043456160] [PMID: 14754413]

[43] Song H, Wang G, He B, *et al.* Cationic lipid-coated PEI/DNA polyplexes with improved efficiency and reduced cytotoxicity for gene delivery into mesenchymal stem cells. Int J Nanomedicine 2012; 7: 4637-48. [PMID: 22942645]

[44] Martin B, Sainlos M, Aissaoui A, *et al.* The design of cationic lipids for gene delivery. Curr Pharm Des 2005; 11(3): 375-94. [http://dx.doi.org/10.2174/1381612053382133] [PMID: 15723632]

[45] Hsu SH, Yu B, Wang X, *et al.* Cationic lipid nanoparticles for therapeutic delivery of siRNA and

miRNA to murine liver tumor. Nanomedicine (Lond) 2013; 9(8): 1169-80. [http://dx.doi.org/10.1016/j.nano.2013.05.007] [PMID: 23727126]

[46] Zhang M, Zhou X, Wang B, Yung B, Lee L, Ghoshal K, *et al.* Lactosylated Gramicidin-based lipid nanoparticles (Lac-GLN) for targeted delivery of anti-miR-155 to hepatocellular carcinoma. J Control Release Soc 2013; 168.

[47] Pramanik D, Campbell NR, Karikari C, Chivukula R, Kent OA, Mendell JT, *et al.* Restitution of tumor suppressor microRNAs using a systemic nanovector inhibits pancreatic cancer growth in mice. Mol Cancer Ther 2011; 10(8): 1470-80. [http://dx.doi.org/10.1158/1535-7163.MCT-11-0152] [PMID: 21622730]

[48] Wu Y, Crawford M, Mao Y, *et al.* Therapeutic delivery of MicroRNA-29b by cationic lipoplexes for lung cancer. Mol Ther Nucleic Acids 2013; 2(4): e84. [http://dx.doi.org/10.1038/mtna.2013.14] [PMID: 23591808]

[49] Piao L, Zhang M, Datta J, Xie X, Su T, Li H, *et al.* Lipid-based nanoparticle delivery of Pre-miR-107 inhibits the tumorigenicity of head and neck squamous cell carcinoma. Molecular Therapy: J Americ Soc Gene Therapy 2012; 20(6): 1261-9. [http://dx.doi.org/10.1038/mt.2012.67] [PMID: 22491216]

[50] Liu XQ, Song WJ, Sun TM, Zhang PZ, Wang J. Targeted delivery of antisense inhibitor of miRNA for antiangiogenesis therapy using cRGD-functionalized nanoparticles. Mol Pharm 2011; 8(1): 250-9. [http://dx.doi.org/10.1021/mp100315q] [PMID: 21138272]

[51] Endo-Takahashi Y, Negishi Y, Nakamura A, *et al.* Systemic delivery of miR-126 by miRNA-loaded Bubble liposomes for the treatment of hindlimb ischemia. Sci Rep 2014; 4: 3883. [http://dx.doi.org/10.1038/srep03883] [PMID: 24457599]

[52] Zhang Q, Ran R, Zhang L, Liu Y, Mei L, Zhang Z, *et al.* Simultaneous delivery of therapeutic antagomirs with paclitaxel for the management of metastatic tumors by a pH-responsive anti-microbial peptide-mediated liposomal delivery system. Journal of controlled release : official journal of the Controlled Release Society. 2015 Jan 10;197:208-18. PubMed PMID: 25445692. Epub 2014/12/03. eng. [http://dx.doi.org/10.1016/j.jconrel.2014.11.010]

[53] Fernandez-Piñeiro I, Badiola I, Sanchez A. Nanocarriers for microRNA delivery in cancer medicine. Biotechnol Adv 2017; 35(3): 350-60. [http://dx.doi.org/10.1016/j.biotechadv.2017.03.002] [PMID: 28286148]

[54] Oh B, Song H, Lee D, *et al.* Anti-cancer effect of R3V6 peptide-mediated delivery of an anti-microRNA-21 antisense-oligodeoxynucleotide in a glioblastoma animal model. J Drug Target 2017; 25(2): 132-9. [http://dx.doi.org/10.1080/1061186X.2016.1207648] [PMID: 27355932]

[55] Song H, Oh B, Choi M, Oh J, Lee M. Delivery of anti-microRNA-21 antisense-oligodeoxynucleotide using amphiphilic peptides for glioblastoma gene therapy. J Drug Target 2015; 23(4): 360-70. [http://dx.doi.org/10.3109/1061186X.2014.1000336] [PMID: 25572456]

[56] Suh JS, Lee JY, Choi YS, Chung CP, Park YJ. Peptide-mediated intracellular delivery of miRNA-29b for osteogenic stem cell differentiation. Biomaterials 2013; 34(17): 4347-59. [http://dx.doi.org/10.1016/j.biomaterials.2013.02.039] [PMID: 23478036]

[57] Schnittert J, Kuninty PR, Bystry TF, Brock R, Storm G, Prakash J. Anti-microRNA targeting using peptide-based nanocomplexes to inhibit differentiation of human pancreatic stellate cells. Nanomedicine (Lond) 2017; 12(12): 1369-84. [http://dx.doi.org/10.2217/nnm-2017-0054] [PMID: 28524768]

[58] Wang KY, McCurdy S, Shea RG, Swaminathan S, Bolton PH. A DNA aptamer which binds to and inhibits thrombin exhibits a new structural motif for DNA. Biochemistry 1993; 32(8): 1899-904. [http://dx.doi.org/10.1021/bi00059a003] [PMID: 8448147]

[59] Dai F, Zhang Y, Zhu X, Shan N, Chen Y. Anticancer role of MUC1 aptamer-miR-29b chimera in epithelial ovarian carcinoma cells through regulation of PTEN methylation. Target Oncol 2012; 7(4): 217-25.
[http://dx.doi.org/10.1007/s11523-012-0236-7] [PMID: 23179556]

[60] Binzel DW, Shu Y, Li H, Sun M, Zhang Q, Shu D, *et al.* Specific Delivery of MiRNA for High Efficient Inhibition of Prostate Cancer by RNA Nanotechnology. Molecular therapy : the journal of the American Society of Gene Therapy. 2016 Aug;24(7):1267-77. PubMed PMID: 27125502. Pubmed Central PMCID: PMC5088763. Epub 2016/04/30. eng.
[http://dx.doi.org/10.1038/mt.2016.85]

[61] Shu D, Li H, Shu Y, *et al.* Systemic Delivery of Anti-miRNA for Suppression of Triple Negative Breast Cancer Utilizing RNA Nanotechnology. ACS Nano 2015; 9(10): 9731-40.
[http://dx.doi.org/10.1021/acsnano.5b02471] [PMID: 26387848]

[62] Iaboni M, Russo V, Fontanella R, *et al.* Aptamer-miRNA-212 Conjugate Sensitizes NSCLC Cells to TRAIL. Mol Ther Nucleic Acids 2016; 5(3): e289.
[http://dx.doi.org/10.1038/mtna.2016.5] [PMID: 27111415]

[63] Tanno T, Zhang P, Lazarski CA, Liu Y, Zheng P. An aptamer-based targeted delivery of miR-26a protects mice against chemotherapy toxicity while suppressing tumor growth. Blood Adv 2017 Jun 27; 1(15): 1107-19.
[http://dx.doi.org/10.1182/bloodadvances.2017004705] [PMID: 29296753]

[64] Baker A, Saltik M, Lehrmann H, *et al.* Polyethylenimine (PEI) is a simple, inexpensive and effective reagent for condensing and linking plasmid DNA to adenovirus for gene delivery. Gene Ther 1997; 4(8): 773-82.
[http://dx.doi.org/10.1038/sj.gt.3300471] [PMID: 9338005]

[65] Biray Avcı Ç, Özcan İ, Balcı T, Özer Ö, Gündüz C. Design of polyethylene glycol-polyethylenimine nanocomplexes as non-viral carriers: mir-150 delivery to chronic myeloid leukemia cells. Cell Biol Int 2013; 37(11): 1205-14.
[http://dx.doi.org/10.1002/cbin.10157] [PMID: 23881828]

[66] Hwang DW, Son S, Jang J, *et al.* A brain-targeted rabies virus glycoprotein-disulfide linked PEI nanocarrier for delivery of neurogenic microRNA. Biomaterials 2011; 32(21): 4968-75.
[http://dx.doi.org/10.1016/j.biomaterials.2011.03.047] [PMID: 21489620]

[67] Yang YP, Chien Y, Chiou GY, *et al.* Inhibition of cancer stem cell-like properties and reduced chemoradioresistance of glioblastoma using microRNA145 with cationic polyurethane-short branch PEI. Biomaterials 2012; 33(5): 1462-76.
[http://dx.doi.org/10.1016/j.biomaterials.2011.10.071] [PMID: 22098779]

[68] Ibrahim AF, Weirauch U, Thomas M, Grünweller A, Hartmann RK, Aigner A. MicroRNA replacement therapy for miR-145 and miR-33a is efficacious in a model of colon carcinoma. Cancer Res 2011; 71(15): 5214-24.
[http://dx.doi.org/10.1158/0008-5472.CAN-10-4645] [PMID: 21690566]

[69] Huang Z, Shi T, Zhou Q, *et al.* miR-141 Regulates colonic leukocytic trafficking by targeting CXCL12β during murine colitis and human Crohn's disease. Gut 2014; 63(8): 1247-57.
[http://dx.doi.org/10.1136/gutjnl-2012-304213] [PMID: 24000293]

[70] Shi T, Xie Y, Fu Y, *et al.* The signaling axis of microRNA-31/interleukin-25 regulates Th1/Th17-mediated inflammation response in colitis. Mucosal Immunol 2017; 10(4): 983-95.
[http://dx.doi.org/10.1038/mi.2016.102] [PMID: 27901018]

[71] Wu LP, Ficker M, Christensen JB, Trohopoulos PN, Moghimi SM. Dendrimers in medicine: therapeutic concepts and pharmaceutical challenges. Bioconjug Chem 2015; 26(7): 1198-211.
[http://dx.doi.org/10.1021/acs.bioconjchem.5b00031] [PMID: 25654320]

[72] Liu X, Li G, Su Z, *et al.* Poly(amido amine) is an ideal carrier of miR-7 for enhancing gene silencing

effects on the EGFR pathway in U251 glioma cells. Oncol Rep 2013; 29(4): 1387-94. [http://dx.doi.org/10.3892/or.2013.2283] [PMID: 23404538]

[73] Ren Y, Kang CS, Yuan XB, *et al.* Co-delivery of as-miR-21 and 5-FU by poly(amidoamine) dendrimer attenuates human glioma cell growth in vitro. J Biomater Sci Polym Ed 2010; 21(3): 303-14. [http://dx.doi.org/10.1163/156856209X415828] [PMID: 20178687]

[74] Gray WD, Wu RJ, Yin X, Zhou J, Davis ME, Luo Y. Dendrimeric bowties featuring hemispheric-selective decoration of ligands for microRNA-based therapy. Biomacromolecules 2013; 14(1): 101-9. [http://dx.doi.org/10.1021/bm301393z] [PMID: 23145944]

[75] Wang F, Zhang B, Zhou L, *et al.* Imaging Dendrimer-Grafted Graphene Oxide Mediated Anti-miR-21 Delivery With an Activatable Luciferase Reporter. ACS Appl Mater Interfaces 2016; 8(14): 9014-21. [http://dx.doi.org/10.1021/acsami.6b02662] [PMID: 27010367]

[76] Blum JS, Saltzman WM. High loading efficiency and tunable release of plasmid DNA encapsulated in submicron particles fabricated from PLGA conjugated with poly-L-lysine. J Control Release Soc 2008; 129(1): 66-72. [http://dx.doi.org/10.1016/j.jconrel.2008.04.002] [PMID: 18511145]

[77] Kulkarni RK, Moore EG, Hegyeli AF, Leonard F. Biodegradable poly(lactic acid) polymers. J Biomed Mater Res 1971; 5(3): 169-81. [http://dx.doi.org/10.1002/jbm.820050305] [PMID: 5560994]

[78] Uchegbu IF. Pharmaceutical nanotechnology: polymeric vesicles for drug and gene delivery. Expert Opin Drug Deliv 2006; 3(5): 629-40. [http://dx.doi.org/10.1517/17425247.3.5.629] [PMID: 16948558]

[79] Devulapally R, Sekar NM, Sekar TV, *et al.* Polymer nanoparticles mediated codelivery of antimiR-10b and antimiR-21 for achieving triple negative breast cancer therapy. ACS Nano 2015; 9(3): 2290-302. [http://dx.doi.org/10.1021/nn507465d] [PMID: 25652012]

[80] Wang S, Zhang J, Wang Y, Chen M. Hyaluronic acid-coated PEI-PLGA nanoparticles mediated co-delivery of doxorubicin and miR-542-3p for triple negative breast cancer therapy. Nanomedicine (Lond) 2016; 12(2): 411-20. [http://dx.doi.org/10.1016/j.nano.2015.09.014] [PMID: 26711968]

[81] Bhargava-Shah A, Foygel K, Devulapally R, Paulmurugan R. Orlistat and antisense-miRNA-loaded PLGA-PEG nanoparticles for enhanced triple negative breast cancer therapy. Nanomedicine (Lond) 2016; 11(3): 235-47. [http://dx.doi.org/10.2217/nnm.15.193] [PMID: 26787319]

[82] Saraiva C, Paiva J, Santos T, Ferreira L, Bernardino L. MicroRNA-124 loaded nanoparticles enhance brain repair in Parkinson's disease. J Control Release Soc 2016; 235: 291-305. [http://dx.doi.org/10.1016/j.jconrel.2016.06.005] [PMID: 27269730]

[83] Tejashri G, Amrita B, Darshana J. Cyclodextrin based nanosponges for pharmaceutical use: a review. Acta Pharm 2013; 63(3): 335-58. [http://dx.doi.org/10.2478/acph-2013-0021] [PMID: 24152895]

[84] Zeng Y, Zhou Z, Fan M, Gong T, Zhang Z, Sun X. PEGylated cationic vectors containing a protease-sensitive peptide as a mirna delivery system for treating breast cancer. Mol Pharm 2017; 14(1): 81-92. [http://dx.doi.org/10.1021/acs.molpharmaceut.6b00726] [PMID: 28043137]

[85] Zuker M. Mfold web server for nucleic acid folding and hybridization prediction. Nucleic Acids Res 2003; 31: 3406-15. [http://dx.doi.org/10.1093/nar/gkg595]

[86] Markham NR, Zuker M. UNAFold: software for nucleic acid folding and hybridization. Methods Mol Biol 2008; 453: 3-31.

[http://dx.doi.org/10.1007/978-1-60327-429-6_1] [PMID: 18712296]

[87] Bindewald E, Grunewald C, Boyle B, O'Connor M, Shapiro BA. Computational strategies for the automated design of RNA nanoscale structures from building blocks using NanoTiler. J Mol Graph Model 2008; 27(3): 299-308.
[http://dx.doi.org/10.1016/j.jmgm.2008.05.004] [PMID: 18838281]

[88] Yingling YG, Shapiro BA. Computational design of an RNA hexagonal nanoring and an RNA nanotube. Nano Lett 2007; 7(8): 2328-34.
[http://dx.doi.org/10.1021/nl070984r] [PMID: 17616164]

[89] Afonin KA, Bindewald E, Yaghoubian AJ, Voss N, Jacovetty E, Shapiro BA, *et al. In vitro* assembly of cubic RNA-based scaffolds designed in silico. Nat Nanotechnol 2010; 5(9): 676-82.
[PMID: 20802494]

[90] Watts JK, Deleavey GF, Damha MJ. Chemically modified siRNA: tools and applications. Drug Discov Today 2008; 13(19-20): 842-55.
[http://dx.doi.org/10.1016/j.drudis.2008.05.007] [PMID: 18614389]

[91] Mathé C, Périgaud C. Cheminform abstract: recent approaches in the synthesis of conformationally restricted nucleoside analogues. European J Organic Chem 2008; 2008: 1489-505.

[92] Liu J, Guo S, Cinier M, *et al.* Fabrication of stable and RNase-resistant RNA nanoparticles active in gearing the nanomotors for viral DNA packaging. ACS Nano 2011; 5(1): 237-46.
[http://dx.doi.org/10.1021/nn1024658] [PMID: 21155596]

[93] Prabha S, Zhou WZ, Panyam J, Labhasetwar V. Size-dependency of nanoparticle-mediated gene transfection: studies with fractionated nanoparticles. Int J Pharm 2002; 244(1-2): 105-15.
[http://dx.doi.org/10.1016/S0378-5173(02)00315-0] [PMID: 12204570]

[94] Abdelmawla S, Guo S, Zhang L, Pulukuri SM, Patankar P, Conley P, *et al.* Pharmacological characterization of chemically synthesized monomeric phi29 pRNA nanoparticles for systemic delivery. Molecular Therapy: J American Soc of Gene Therapy 2011; 19(7): 1312-22.
[http://dx.doi.org/10.1038/mt.2011.35] [PMID: 21468004]

[95] Sioud M. RNA therapeutics: function, design, and delivery. Preface. Methods Mol Biol 2010; 629: v-vii.
[http://dx.doi.org/10.1007/978-1-60761-657-3] [PMID: 20394129]

[96] Jasinski DL, Schwartz CT, Haque F, Guo P. Large scale purification of RNA nanoparticles by preparative ultracentrifugation. Methods Mol Biol 2015; 1297: 67-82.
[http://dx.doi.org/10.1007/978-1-4939-2562-9_5] [PMID: 25895996]

[97] Cui D, Zhang C, Liu B, Shu Y, Du T, Shu D, *et al.* Regression of gastric cancer by systemic injection of rna nanoparticles carrying both ligand and siRNA. Scientific Rep 2015; 5: 10726.
[http://dx.doi.org/10.1038/srep10726]

[98] Guo S, Tschammer N, Mohammed S, Guo P. Specific delivery of therapeutic RNAs to cancer cells via the dimerization mechanism of phi29 motor pRNA. Hum Gene Ther 2005; 16(9): 1097-109.
[http://dx.doi.org/10.1089/hum.2005.16.1097] [PMID: 16149908]

[99] Kwon YJ. Before and after endosomal escape: roles of stimuli-converting siRNA/polymer interactions in determining gene silencing efficiency. Acc Chem Res 2012; 45(7): 1077-88.
[http://dx.doi.org/10.1021/ar200241v] [PMID: 22103667]

CHAPTER 9

Nanoparticle Immunotherapy

Abstract: Immunostimulatory agents such as adjuvants, cytokines, and antibodies have a great potential for the treatment of disease conditions. However, their direct administration may lead to suboptimal pharmacokinetics, compromised targeting and vulnerability to biodegradation. To overcome these drawbacks, nanoparticles play a vital role and they improve the delivery mechanism of these therapeutic agents. The nanoparticle in conjugation elevates the bioavailability of the encapsulated payloads. In this study, we intended to discuss these immunostimulants when delivered by nanoparticles.

Keywords: Adjuvant, Antibody, Antigens, Breast cancer, Cytokines, Dendritic cells, Dextran nanoparticle, Gold nanoparticle, Immunostimulants, Immunosuppression, Inorganic nanoparticle, Lipid nanoparticle, Melanoma, Mesoporous silica nanoparticle, Microenvironment, Organic nanoparticle, OVA, PEG, PLGA, Polymeric nanoparticle, Toll like receptor.

INTRODUCTION

The immune system is composed of different types of specialized immune cells that are highly efficient at eliminating foreign particles. Recently, a variety of nanoparticles in conjugation with wide variety of drugs have developed that helped in clinical diagnosis and therapy. These nanoparticles include inorganic, organic and polymeric types that help in the delivery of therapeutic and diagnostic agents [1]. Nanoparticles help in the delivery of cancer specific drugs that increases their efficacy that results into increased safety and prolongs circulation time and bioavailability [2]. Therefore, nanoparticles have gained increased interest by the researchers in drug delivery and diagnostics.

Generally, the immune modulators when administered in solution produce many adverse side effects and toxicity, but when they are introduced within the systemic circulation in conjugation with nanoparticles, they may overcome many adverse side effects. In this study, we intended to discuss the wide variety of antigens, adjuvants, *etc.* when delivered by nanoparticles in conjugation as an immunotherapy.

Rituparna Acharya

NANOPARTICLES IN IMMUNOTHERAPY

Antigen Delivery by Nanoparticles

Over the soluble formulations when antigens are loaded in a nanoparticle, they demonstrate special advantages. Firstly, when antigens are encapsulated within the nanoparticles, they protect them from proteolysis degradation. Secondly, the nanoconjugates are restricted from entering in to the systemic circulation and they increase the localized dosages. Lastly, nanoconjugates help the dendritic cells to cross-present the antigens more efficiently than bare antigens [3].

In one publication, Gao *et al.*, formulated carboxymethyl chitosan/chitosan nanoparticles (CMCS/CS-NPs) in conjugation with extracellular products (ECPs) of *Vibrio anguillarum* that exhibited greater innate and adaptive immune response [4]. Another study investigated the property of cationic liposomes on the antigen presentation andmaturation of dendritic cells. Greater efficiency was demonstrated by the cationic liposomes on activation of dendritic cells and antigen presentation to T cells by antigen presenting cells [5]. When Rietscher *et al.*, conjugated the model ovalbumin (OVA) with hydrophilic polyethyleneglycol (PEG)-b-PAGE-b-poly(lactic-co-glycolic acid) (PPP), they discovered that *in vitro* activation of T cells by antigen presenting cells increased significantly in comparison with soluble and free OVA antigen [6].

Adjuvant Delivery by Nanoparticles

Adjuvants are the moieties that mimic pathogen associated molecular patterns (PAMPs) such as bacterial cell wall components *e.g.* mannose, lipopolysaccharides (LPS) and nucleic acids [7]. When these adjuvants are in conjunction with antigens, they greatly boost the activities of lymphocytes, dendritic cells and macrophages. But these immunostimulators may produce side effects for example toxic shock syndrome in many cases [8, 9]. In this regard, nanoparticles may reduce the toxic side effects of the aforementioned adjuvant by their unique property [10].

One of the types of adjuvant is oligonucleotides with CpG island binding with the Toll-like receptor (TLR)-9 of the dendritic cells and stimulating them [11]. However, when they are loaded in a cationic gelatin-based nanoparticle, it activates dendritic cells, antigen presenting cells, and T lymphocyte. Moreover, it develops protective anti-tumor immunity in the mouse model of melanoma [12, 13].

Schlosser *et al.*, demonstrated that cytotoxic T lymphocyte responses were enhanced when OVA model adjuvant was encapsulated within a PLGA nanoparticle in comparison with a soluble adjuvant [14]. Moreover, in PLGA nanoparticle when tyrosinase-related protein 2 (TRP2), poorly immunogenic melanoma antigen, along with adjuvant monophosphoryl lipid A were co-delivered, they showed therapeutic antitumor effect [15]. In a study, when autophagosomes derived from tumor cells or model tumor antigen were delivered through α-Al_2O_3 nanoparticle, they resulted in tumor regression [16]. Another study reported polymeric nanoparticle when coated with layer of cancer membranes could promote a tumor antigen specific immune response [17].

Co-delivery of Antigen and Adjuvant by Nanoparticles

Co-delivery of antigen and adjutants together has the potential to develop immune response to the target cell. Recently, a publication discussed the delivery of toll-like receptor 3 (TLR3) agonist and protein tumor antigen (OVA) by the nanoparticle poly(γ-glutamic acid) (γ-PGA) based SVNPs that have enhanced the anti-tumor immunity in mice model [18]. In another study, pyruvate dehydrogenase E2 protein nanoparticle used for the delivery of CpG and gp100 melanoma-associated epitope increased the proliferation of CD8+ T-cells and Type II interferon IFN-γ secretion [19].

Activation of Dendritic Cells by Nanoparticles

Actively targeting dendritic cells may be a future therapeutic application for several disease conditions [20]. Nanoparticles tagged with the legend of the receptors on dendritic cells demonstrated improved nanoparticle uptake by the cell through receptor mediated endocytosis *in vivo* [21, 22]. There are several dendritic cell surface ligands such as fucose N-acetyl glucosamine, mannose, anti-DEC205and anti-CD11c. By binding of nanoparticles with these ligands significantly improve the activation of dendritic cells. Kempf *et al.* fabricated PLGA nanoparticles that target the ligands of the dendritic cell surface molecule [21]. In the formulation of vaccine Kranz *et al.* evidenced that dendritic cells may be targeted with RNA-lipoplexes increases the efficacy *in vivo* [23]. A nanovaccine was functionalized using tumor antigen peptides (TAPs) that targeted the dendritic cells *via* the scavenger receptor class B1 (SRB1) ligand pathway [24]. However, it has been studied that large particles with a size range of 500–2000 nm gets into the lymph nodes after the uptake by the dendritic cells, on the other hand small nanoparticles with a range of 20–200 nm may target the dendritic cells within the lymph nodes and may drain freely to the lymph nodes [25]. In future, detail study is need of the hour for eliciting dendritic cell manipulation [26].

Change of Tumor Microenvironment by Nanoparticles

Tumor microenvironment has several properties that complicate the immunotherapy through nanoparticles. The properties include irregular vascularization, low extracellular pH, hypoxic conditions, and enhanced proteolytic activities [27]. Moreover, tumor microenvironment produces a immunosuppressive condition by wide variety of mechanisms. Nanoparticles targeting towards the immunosuppressive cells such as myeloid-derived suppressive cells (MDSCs), tumor-associated macrophages (TAMs) and regulatory T cells (Tregs)offer a potential treatment procedure for cancer [28].

In one study Park *et al.* formulated nanolipogels (nLGs) conjugated with cyclodextrins and polymers that encapsulate the cytokine [29]. This nanoconjugate may deliver the IL-2 and an inhibitor of TGF-β that delayed in tumor growth, activated of natural killer (NK) cells and activation of CD8+ cytotoxic T lymphocytes. PEG modified single-walled carbon nanotubes (PEG-SWCNTs) was developed in conjugation with glucocorticoid-induced TNFR-related receptor [30]. Another study targeted TAM by using PEG-sheddable, mannose-modified nanoparticles [31]. Chemotherapeutic application has remodeled the microenvironment and improved the immunotherapy [32]. Combination therapy of a curcumin-PEG (CUR-PEG) micelle and a TRP2 antigen resulted into antitumor effect in melanoma mice model [33].Wang *et al.* demonstrated that after the injection of PEG-SWCNTs it modulate adaptive immune responses and specifically the cellular immunity of metastatic cancer [34].

Delivery of Antibodics by Nanoparticlcs

The antibodies when used as therapeutic measure they face certain limitations such as less interactions with the immune system, impaired pharmacokinetics and less tissue accessibility. To overcome these limitations nanoparticles are used as a therapeutic measure [35]. In a study polyion complex micelles (PICs) was loaded with homo- and block-catiomers in antibody enhanced the endosomal escape efficacy and enhanced the recognition of intracellular antigens [36]. When, anti-OX40 antibody was loaded onto a PLGAnanoparticle it induced cytotoxic T lymphocyte proliferation, cytokine production and tumor antigen-specific cytotoxicity in an enhanced level than free anti-OX40 antibody [37]. Further, when CTLA-4 antibody was functionalized mesoporous silica (FMS) it induced a much enhanced and extended therapeutic response [38].

Co-delivery of antibody and cytokines through nanoparticles demonstrated promising results in recent publications. For example when anti-CD137 antibody and IL-2Fc protein was conjugated with PEGylated liposomes murine B16F10 model it avoided the toxicities caused by soluble immunotherapy and produced antitumor memory [39]. Another study showed the effect of alginate hydrogel system for delivering celecoxib and PD-1 antibody to treat tumor-bearing mice [40]. It enhanced the antitumor activity when used in combination. In a study when nanoparticle was used to deliver anti-PD-L1 antibody and anti-4-1BB51 antibody it caused a 6-fold enhanced IFN-γ production by CD8+ T cells and alsodecrease in tumor infiltrating lymphocytes [41].

Gene Delivery by Nanoparticles

siRNA delivery as a part of gene therapy may have effective property of immunostimulation through nanoparticles. When lipid-assisted PEG–PLGA-based nanoparticle delivering CTLA-4 siRNA showed effectively internalization within the T cells and enhanced T cell proliferation. Moreover, the systemic delivery of the nanoconjugate significantly enhanced the proliferation of CD4+ T cells and CD8+ T cells, inhibited tumor growth, and prolonged the survival of mice melanoma model [42]. When polymer is conjugated with folic acid and PD-L1 siRNAit leads to the rapid uptake of the conjugate by SKOV-3-luc cells. This condition inhibits the non-specific uptake by monocytes [43]. Moreover, when PD-L1 and PD-L2 siRNAs were delivered using cationic amphiphilic lipid SAINT-18 (1-methyl-4-(cis-9-dioleyl)methyl-pyridinium-chloride) and dioleoyl phosphatidyl ethanolamine then the knockdown of PD-L was achieved without effecting dendritic cell viability or maturation [44].When, TGF-β siRNA was using through liposome-protamine-hyaluronic acid nanoparticle it resulted in TGF-β down-regulation that inhibited tumor growth due to enhanced tumor infiltration by CD8+ T cells [45].

Cytokine Delivery by Nanoparticles

Cytokines have special ability to stimulate immune response, so they are approved by FDA for cancer immunotherapy. For proper therapeutic effect cytokines leads to rapid degradation and excretion. To overcome these limitations high dose of cytokines are necessary, but this results into toxic side effects [46]. In this respect nanoparticles plays a vital role that have no side effects. In a study stealth liposomes are used to deliver IL-2. The resultant nanoconjugate significantly reduced tumor growth in mice model with advanced metastatic lung cancer [47]. A study was conducted on advanced solid tumor treated by PEGylated liposome encapsulating TNF-α [48]. A study on follicular lymphoma was conducted, where it was treated IL-2 and a TAA demonstrated increased tumor infiltration by lymphocytes and regressed tumor growth [49]. A wide variety of cytokines including IL-1a, IL-2, IL-6 or GM-CSF may be delivered using liposomes that have future in therapeutics [50].

Therapeutic Cellular Engineering by Nanoparticles

In cellular engineering T cells and (HSCs) were conjugated with liposomes and lipid-coated PLGA nanoparticles in a range of diameter 100-300 nm was used to target antigen-expressing tumors [51]. A therapeutic cargo was constructed using TWS119 – a glycogen synthase kinase-3 β (GSK-3β) inhibitor encapsulated within multilamellar lipid nanoparticle demonstrated a slow release period up to seven days and thus enhancing the hematopoietic stem cell HSCs reconstitution [52]. In a study PLGA nanoparticle was conjugated with melanoma or prostate tumor cells and TLR9-ligand with CpG that activated dendritic cells to trigger anti-tumor immuneresponses. For cancer immunotherapy, a study was designed with polystyrene nanoparticle in conjugation with multivalent bi-specific nanobioconjugate engager (mBiNE) and with anti-HER2 antibody and calreticulin [53]. The main advantages of mBiNE method are for example it promotes phagocytosis of cancer cells by activation of macrophages. Secondly, enhanced activation of antigen presenting cells. Thirdly, activation of antitumor immune responses *in vivo* and lastly, formation of durable and systemic antitumorimmunity.The mechanism of action of the mBiNE in case of cancer immunotherapy is *via* T-cell activation, phagocytosis and immune-inducedcytotoxic killing.

Overcoming Immunosuppression by Nanoparticles

To modulate antitumor immune response immune checkpoint molecules are used that are involved in the regulation of T-cell [54]. The cytotoxic T-lymphocyt--associated antigen 4 (CTLA4) that are expressed onactivated T-cells, and the programmed cell death protein 1 (PD1) that may bind to ligands such as PD-L1 and PD-L2, are widely being utilized for this purpose [55 - 57]. To restore antitumor immunity anti-CTLA4 antibody drug, for example Ipilimumab and anti-PD1 antibody drugs such as Durvalumab, Nivolumab, Pembrolizumab and Atezolizumab are approved for clinical uses. However, the antibody based immunotherapy have drawback such as non-specific antibody accumulation in the cells may produce toxicity [58].

Immune Check Point Inhibition by Nanoparticles

Cancer immunotherapy may address the immune check point inhibition by using nanoparticles. A nanoparticle was fabricated using poly (ethylene glycol) 5000---poly (D,L-lactide) 11000 (PEG-PLA) copolymer, and siCTLA4 siRNA with N-bis (2-hydroxyethly)-N-methyl-N-(2-cholestery loxycarbony laminoethyl) ammonium bromide (BHEM-Chol) that was encapsulated within the PEG-PLA nanoparticles [59]. This polymeric nanoconjugateinterferes with immune suppression and they increase both CD4+ T-cells and CD8+ T-cells, on the other hand CD4+ FOXP3+ regulatory T-cells were decreased in number that leads to theinhibition of tumor growth and prolonged survival of B16 mouse melanoma model.PD-L1 may be used as an attractive target for immune checkpoint modulation as they are expressed in various tumor cells [60] including melanoma [61, 62], ovarian cancer [63], non-small cell lungcancer [64], head and neck cancer [65], thymic cancer [66] and B-cell lymphoma [67]. Another publication showed efficiently inhibited by PD-L1 siRNA on SKOV-3-Luc tumor cells when they are conjugated with folic acid-modified PEI, leads to sensitizing tumor cells to T-cell killing *in vitro* [43]. When anti-PD-L1 antibody was conjugated with platelets that helped to enhance the efficacy ofdelivery of anti-PDL1 that results into the reduction of rick in cancer re-occurrence and metastatic spreading *in vitro* and *in vivo* [68]. Further, another immune modulation strategy is direct delivery of immune modulating compounds to the CD8+ T-cells in conjugation with nanoparticle delivery vehicle [69, 70]. For example, anti-PD1 antibody was conjugated with poly (ethylene glycol)-poly (lactic-co-glycolic acid) (PEG-PLGA) nanoparticle. Co-delivery of Resiquimod (R848) or SD-208, transforming growth factor β (TGF β) inhibitors, along with anti-PD1 fragments-conjugated with PEG-PLGA nanoparticle leads to *in vivo* T-cell targeting [71].

Recently, the anticancer drugs and/or immunecheckpoint inhibitors were developed that may be administered transdermally by using self-degradable microneedle (MN) patches when they are conjugated with nanoparticles [72, 73].

Induced Immunogenic Cell Death by Nanoparticles

It has been demonstrated that the apoptotic tumor cells may elicit an immune response by releasing damage-associated molecular patterns (DAMPs), this leads to the trigger of an anti-tumor effect during photodynamic therapies, chemotherapies, photothermal therapies and radiotherapies [74 - 77]. As a result of immunogenic cell death (ICD) in the tumor, immune activation occurs.Moreover, the translocation of calreticulin (CRT) on the cell surface leads to the release of high-mobility group box 1 (HMGB1) protein and ATP [78, 79]. Further, the activated antigen presenting cells and the activation of CD8+ cytotoxic T lymphocytes after phagocytosis of dying tumor cells, the dendritic cells may lead to activation of adaptive immune system. After this discovery, the immuno therapies has been investigated using immune checkpoint inhibitors [80], vaccines [81], adoptive cell transfer (ACT) [82] and anthracycline chemodrugs [83].

Wide variety of nanoparticles have been discovered for the various types of co-delivery of ICD inducers and immune adjuvants for the enhancement of anti-tumor immunotherapy response. The nanoparticles such as poly(lactic-coglycolic acid) (PLGA) have been utilized to activate the ICD by the delivery of doxorubicin (DOX) and CpG oligodeoxynucleotides at the tumor site [84]. In pancreatic tumor animal model monomethoxypoly (ethylene glycol)-modified PLGA nanoparticle was used to encapsulate oxaliplatin *i.e.,* an ICD inducer orgemcitabine *i.e.,* a non-ICD inducer may increase ICD effect and the cytotoxic effect of the tumor [85]. Another nanoparticle was developed using chitosan-coated hollow copper sulfide that intercalated theCpG (HCuSNPs-CpG) were used for photothermal immunotherapy in breast cancer animal model [86].

TYPES OF NANOPARTICLES IN IMMUNOTHERAPY

Nanoparticles are the materials having size less than 100nm. These particles improve the bioavailability and pharmacokinetics of their pay load. Moreover, they may stimulate after targeting the immune system and thatleads to the production of cytokines that mediate cellular and humoral immunity. In this section we are intended to discus about the variety of nanoparticles that are used for immune modulation and vaccination.

Inorganic Nanoparticles

Among the inorganic nanoparticles, gold nanoparticles are the promising delivery vehicle for their safety and tunable property [87]. Gold nanoparticles may decrease the adverse effect of the immunostimulators when they are delivered in soluble form. In a study when gold nanoparticles are conjugated with a tumor homing peptide that binds to CD13 on tumor endothelium were found to release TNFα *in vivo* [88]. When anti-PD-L1 antibody was conjugated with gold nanoparticle and administered to tumor-bearing mice it produced signal in CT scan that correlated with tumor growth and T cell infiltration [89].

Mesoporous silica nanoparticles are another type of inorganic nanoparticle that has the property of biocompatibility and biodegradability [90, 91]. Due to their porous structure mesoporous silica nanoparticles have high payload carrying capacity. When, liposome-coated mesoporous silica nanoparticles were conjugated with doxorubicin and oxaliplatin along with indoximod *i.e.,* an immunometabolic adjuvant they interfere with immunosuppression in the tumor site [92]. This nanoparticle may be used as a delivery vehicle of TNF α that reduces the dosage [93]. Mesoporous silica nanoparticles when conjugated with photothermal agents and model antigens they are capable of eliciting strong immune responses. Moreover, they generateactivated CD4+ and CD8+ T cells as a combined effect. Further, when glutathione-depleted dendritic mesoporous silica nanoparticles were conjugated with a model antigen and CpG ODN they deliver the payload intra cellularly leading to the generation of reactive oxygen species that further intensify the immune responses [94].

Organic Nanoparticles

Within organic nanoparticles liposomal nanoparticles are highly studied as it have improved biocompatibility and therapeutic potential for immunostimulation. Recently wide varieties of immunostimulants are loaded to the liposomal carrier and studied their advantages. A major hurdle for the use of cytokines and mAbs directly are their systemic toxicity, specifically on lymphocytes. To overcome this hurdle, nanoparticles are been leveraged for passive targeting and carry the payload to the tumor sites [95, 96]. In a study PEGylated liposomes in conjugation with IL2 and anti-CD137 antibody were fabricated that leads to remarkable tumor accumulation and improved antibody localization in comparison with their soluble forms. Further, this formulation delayed the tumor growth without any adverse effect [97].

Polymeric Nanoparticles

Polymeric carriers are the most studied nanoparticles for the delivery of immunostimulatory molecules. They are highly biocompatible and have wide range of encapsulation and conjugation options. Polymeric nanoparticles deliver adjuvant payloads such as R837, encapsulated into a polyethylene glycol (PEG)–poly(lactic-co-glycolic acid) (PLGA) nanoparticle [98]. The use of combine checkpoint inhibitor for the activation of dendritic cells has a potential therapeutic option with promising immunotherapy approach [99]. While the administration of adjutants may directly result in side effects and make them inappropriate for the treatment of disease conditions. To overcome the adverse effects, nanoparticles are fabricated such as block copolymer comprising of methoxy triethylene glycol methacrylate and penta fluorophenyl methacrylate and been functionalized with TLR7/8 agonists that are capable of activating dendritic cells in the tumor site [100]. Moreover, OX40 antibody was conjugated with PLGA nanoparticles demonstrating the advantages of the nanoparticulate formulation [101].

Acetalated dextran has been demonstrated as a good material for cancer immunotherapies [102] This nanoparticle has higher efficiency of loading hydrophilic drugs that made them a better option for carrying the payload [103]. In a study, it has been demonstrated that acetalated dextran microparticles encapsulated CpG ODN more efficiently than PLGA nanoparticles [104].

CONCLUSION

Immune therapy using nanoparticles helps in effective immunostimulation with long lasting immune response. This approach is found to be more effective than non-nanoparticle based therapy. In order to get high efficiency and low toxicity, fabrication of efficient nanoparticle is the need of the hour. The nanoparticles should have the properties such as pharmacokinetics, high stability, efficient biodistribution and low toxicity. The delivery of adjuvants, cytokines, and monoclonal antibodies gets benefited by use in conjugation with nanoparticles. When used in conjugation, it increases the biological activity and bioavailability and leads to stronger immune stimulation.

In this study, we intended to discuss the payloads that need to be delivered to elucidate immunostimulation in long lasting fashion. Moreover, a wide variety of nanoparticles have high efficiency to develop immune responses.

REFERENCES

[1] Kumari P, Ghosh B, Biswas S. Nanocarriers for cancer-targeted drug delivery. J Drug Target 2016; 24(3): 179-91.
[http://dx.doi.org/10.3109/1061186X.2015.1051049] [PMID: 26061298]

[2] Parhi P, Mohanty C, Sahoo SK. Nanotechnology-based combinational drug delivery: an emerging approach for cancer therapy. Drug Discov Today 2012; 17(17-18): 1044-52.
[http://dx.doi.org/10.1016/j.drudis.2012.05.010] [PMID: 22652342]

[3] Fang RH, Kroll AV, Zhang L. Nanoparticle-based manipulation of antigen-presenting cells for cancer immunotherapy. Small (Weinheim an der Bergstrasse, Germany) 2015; 11(41): 5483-96.
[http://dx.doi.org/10.1002/smll.201501284] [PMID: 26331993]

[4] Gao P, Xia G, Bao Z, *et al.* Chitosan based nanoparticles as protein carriers for efficient oral antigen delivery. Int J Biol Macromol 2016; 91: 716-23.
[http://dx.doi.org/10.1016/j.ijbiomac.2016.06.015] [PMID: 27287772]

[5] Maji M, Mazumder S, Bhattacharya S, *et al.* A lipid based antigen delivery system efficiently facilitates mhc class-i antigen presentation in dendritic cells to stimulate CD8(+) T Cells. Sci Rep 2016; 6: 27206.
[http://dx.doi.org/10.1038/srep27206] [PMID: 27251373]

[6] Rietscher R, Schröder M, Janke J, Czaplewska J, Gottschaldt M, Scherließ R, *et al.* Antigen delivery *via* hydrophilic PEG-b-PAGE-b-PLGA nanoparticles boosts vaccination induced T cell immunity. Eur J Pharm Biopharm 2016; 102: 20-31.
[PMID: 26940132]

[7] Gavin AL, Hoebe K, Duong B, *et al.* Adjuvant-enhanced antibody responses in the absence of toll-like receptor signaling. Science 2006; 314(5807): 1936-8.
[http://dx.doi.org/10.1126/science.1135299] [PMID: 17185603]

[8] Shapira L, Soskolne WA, Houri Y, Barak V, Halabi A, Stabholz A. Protection against endotoxic shock and lipopolysaccharide-induced local inflammation by tetracycline: correlation with inhibition of cytokine secretion. Infect Immun 1996; 64(3): 825-8.
[http://dx.doi.org/10.1128/iai.64.3.825-828.1996] [PMID: 8641787]

[9] Gupta RK, Siber GR. Adjuvants for human vaccines--current status, problems and future prospects. Vaccine 1995; 13(14): 1263-76.
[http://dx.doi.org/10.1016/0264-410X(95)00011-O] [PMID: 8585280]

[10] Gutjahr A, Phelip C, Coolen A-L, *et al.* Biodegradable polymeric nanoparticles-based vaccine adjuvants for lymph nodes targeting. Vaccines (Basel) 2016; 4(4): 34.
[http://dx.doi.org/10.3390/vaccines4040034] [PMID: 27754314]

[11] Krieg AM. Therapeutic potential of Toll-like receptor 9 activation. Nat Rev Drug Discov 2006; 5(6): 471-84.
[http://dx.doi.org/10.1038/nrd2059] [PMID: 16763660]

[12] Bourquin C, Anz D, Zwiorek K, Lanz AL, Fuchs S, Weigel S, *et al.* Targeting CpG oligonucleotides to the lymph node by nanoparticles elicits efficient antitumoral immunity. J Immunology (Baltimore, Md : 1950) 2008; 181(5): 2990-8.
[http://dx.doi.org/10.4049/jimmunol.181.5.2990] [PMID: 18713969]

[13] Sokolova V, Knuschke T, Kovtun A, Buer J, Epple M, Westendorf AM. The use of calcium phosphate nanoparticles encapsulating Toll-like receptor ligands and the antigen hemagglutinin to induce dendritic cell maturation and T cell activation. Biomat 2010; 31(21): 5627-33.
[http://dx.doi.org/10.1016/j.biomaterials.2010.03.067]

[14] Schlosser E, Mueller M, Fischer S, *et al.* TLR ligands and antigen need to be coencapsulated into the same biodegradable microsphere for the generation of potent cytotoxic T lymphocyte responses. Vaccine 2008; 26(13): 1626-37.
[http://dx.doi.org/10.1016/j.vaccine.2008.01.030] [PMID: 18295941]

[15] Hamdy S, Molavi O, Ma Z, *et al.* Co-delivery of cancer-associated antigen and Toll-like receptor 4 ligand in PLGA nanoparticles induces potent CD8+ T cell-mediated anti-tumor immunity. Vaccine 2008; 26(39): 5046-57.
[http://dx.doi.org/10.1016/j.vaccine.2008.07.035] [PMID: 18680779]

[16] Li H, Li Y, Jiao J, Hu HM. Alpha-alumina nanoparticles induce efficient autophagy-dependent cross-presentation and potent antitumour response. Nat Nanotechnol 2011; 6(10): 645-50.
[http://dx.doi.org/10.1038/nnano.2011.153] [PMID: 21926980]

[17] Fang RH, Hu C-MJ, Luk BT, Gao W, Copp JA, Tai Y, *et al.* Cancer cell membrane-coated nanoparticles for anticancer vaccination and drug delivery. Nano Letters 2014; 14(4): 2181-8.
[http://dx.doi.org/10.1021/nl500618u]

[18] Kim SY, Noh YW, Kang TH, *et al.* Synthetic vaccine nanoparticles target to lymph node triggering enhanced innate and adaptive antitumor immunity. Biomaterials 2017; 130: 56-66.
[http://dx.doi.org/10.1016/j.biomaterials.2017.03.034] [PMID: 28364631]

[19] Oberli MA, Reichmuth AM, Dorkin JR, *et al.* Lipid nanoparticle assisted mRNA delivery for potent cancer immunotherapy. Nano Lett 2017; 17(3): 1326-35.
[http://dx.doi.org/10.1021/acs.nanolett.6b03329] [PMID: 28273716]

[20] Klippstein R, Pozo D. Nanotechnology-based manipulation of dendritic cells for enhanced immunotherapy strategies. Nanomedicine (Lond) 2010; 6(4): 523-9.
[http://dx.doi.org/10.1016/j.nano.2010.01.001] [PMID: 20085824]

[21] Kempf M, Mandal B, Jilek S, *et al.* Improved stimulation of human dendritic cells by receptor engagement with surface-modified microparticles. J Drug Target 2003; 11(1): 11-8.
[http://dx.doi.org/10.1080/1061186031000072978] [PMID: 12852436]

[22] Dhodapkar MV, Sznol M, Zhao B, *et al.* Induction of antigen-specific immunity with a vaccine targeting NY-ESO-1 to the dendritic cell receptor DEC-205. Sci Transl Med 2014; 6(232): 232ra51.
[http://dx.doi.org/10.1126/scitranslmed.3008068] [PMID: 24739759]

[23] Kranz LM, Diken M, Haas H, *et al.* Systemic RNA delivery to dendritic cells exploits antiviral defence for cancer immunotherapy. Nature 2016; 534(7607): 396-401.
[http://dx.doi.org/10.1038/nature18300] [PMID: 27281205]

[24] Qian Y, Jin H, Qiao S, Dai Y, Huang C, Lu L, *et al.* Targeting dendritic cells in lymph node with an antigen peptide-based nanovaccine for cancer immunotherapy. Biomater 2016; 98: 171-83.
[http://dx.doi.org/10.1016/j.biomaterials.2016.05.008]

[25] Manolova V, Flace A, Bauer M, Schwarz K, Saudan P, Bachmann MF. Nanoparticles target distinct dendritic cell populations according to their size. Eur J Immunol 2008; 38(5): 1404-13.

[http://dx.doi.org/10.1002/eji.200737984] [PMID: 18389478]

[26] Bachmann MF, Jennings GT. Vaccine delivery: a matter of size, geometry, kinetics and molecular patterns. Nat Rev Immunol 2010; 10(11): 787-96. [http://dx.doi.org/10.1038/nri2868] [PMID: 20948547]

[27] Estrella V, Chen T, Lloyd M, *et al.* Acidity generated by the tumor microenvironment drives local invasion. Cancer Res 2013; 73(5): 1524-35. [http://dx.doi.org/10.1158/0008-5472.CAN-12-2796] [PMID: 23288510]

[28] Dunn GP, Old LJ, Schreiber RD. The immunobiology of cancer immunosurveillance and immunoediting. Immunity 2004; 21(2): 137-48. [http://dx.doi.org/10.1016/j.immuni.2004.07.017] [PMID: 15308095]

[29] Park J, Wrzesinski SH, Stern E, *et al.* Combination delivery of TGF-β inhibitor and IL-2 by nanoscale liposomal polymeric gels enhances tumour immunotherapy. Nat Mater 2012; 11(10): 895-905. [http://dx.doi.org/10.1038/nmat3355] [PMID: 22797827]

[30] Sacchetti C, Rapini N, Magrini A, Cirelli E, Bellucci S, Mattei M, *et al. In Vivo* targeting of intratumor regulatory t cells using PEG-modified single-walled carbon nanotubes. Bioconjugate Chem 2013; 24(6): 852-8.

[31] Zhu S, Niu M, O'Mary H, Cui Z. Targeting of tumor-associated macrophages made possible by PEG-sheddable, mannose-modified nanoparticles. Mol Pharm 2013; 10(9): 3525-30. [http://dx.doi.org/10.1021/mp400216r] [PMID: 23901887]

[32] Zhao Y, Huo M, Xu Z, Wang Y, Huang L. Nanoparticle delivery of CDDO-Me remodels the tumor microenvironment and enhances vaccine therapy for melanoma. Biomaterials 2015; 68: 54-66. [http://dx.doi.org/10.1016/j.biomaterials.2015.07.053] [PMID: 26264646]

[33] Lu Y, Miao L, Wang Y, Xu Z, Zhao Y, Shen Y, *et al.* Curcumin micelles remodel tumor microenvironment and enhance vaccine activity in an advanced melanoma model. Molecular Therapy: J American Soc of Gene Therapy 2016; 24(2): 364-74. [http://dx.doi.org/10.1038/mt.2015.165] [PMID: 26334519]

[34] Wang C, Xu L, Liang C, Xiang J, Peng R, Liu Z. Immunological responses triggered by photothermal therapy with carbon nanotubes in combination with anti-CTLA-4 therapy to inhibit cancer metastasis. Adv Mater (Deerfield Beach, Fla). 2014; 26(48): 8154-62. [http://dx.doi.org/10.1002/adma.201402996] [PMID: 25331930]

[35] Elhissi A, Ahmed W, Dhanak VR, Subramani K. Carbon nanotubes in cancer therapy and drug delivery.Emerging Nanotechnologies in Dentistry. Boston: William Andrew Publishing 2012; pp. 347-63. [http://dx.doi.org/10.1016/B978-1-4557-7862-1.00020-1]

[36] Kim A, Miura Y, Ishii T, Mutaf OF, Nishiyama N, Cabral H, *et al.* Intracellular delivery of charge-converted monoclonal antibodies by combinatorial design of block/homo polyion complex micelles. Biomacromol 2016; 17(2): 446-53.

[37] Chen M, Ouyang H, Zhou S, Li J, Ye Y. PLGA-nanoparticle mediated delivery of anti-OX40 monoclonal antibody enhances anti-tumor cytotoxic T cell responses. Cell Immunol 2014; 287(2): 91-9. [http://dx.doi.org/10.1016/j.cellimm.2014.01.003] [PMID: 24487032]

[38] Lei C, Liu P, Chen B, Mao Y, Engelmann H, Shin Y, *et al.* Local Release of Highly Loaded Antibodies from Functionalized Nanoporous Support for Cancer Immunotherapy. J American Chemical Soc 2010; 132(20): 6906-7. [http://dx.doi.org/10.1021/ja102414t]

[39] Kwong B, Gai SA, Elkhader J, Wittrup KD, Irvine DJ. Localized immunotherapy *via* liposome-anchored Anti-CD137 + IL-2 prevents lethal toxicity and elicits local and systemic antitumor immunity. Cancer Res 2013; 73(5): 1547-58.

[http://dx.doi.org/10.1158/0008-5472.CAN-12-3343] [PMID: 23436794]

[40] Li Y, Fang M, Zhang J, *et al.* Hydrogel dual delivered celecoxib and anti-PD-1 synergistically improve antitumor immunity. OncoImmunology 2015; 5(2): e1074374. [http://dx.doi.org/10.1080/2162402X.2015.1074374] [PMID: 27057439]

[41] Kosmides AK, Schneck J. Dual-targeting nanoparticles for reprogrammed T cell responses in the tumor microenvironment. J Immunother Cancer 2014; 2(Suppl 3): P108-P. [PMID: PMC4288393]

[42] Li SY, Liu Y, Xu CF, Shen S, Sun R, Du XJ, *et al.* Restoring anti-tumor functions of T cells *via* nanoparticle-mediated immune checkpoint modulation. J Control Release Soc 2016; 231:17-28. [http://dx.doi.org/10.1016/j.jconrel.2016.01.044] [PMID: 26829099]

[43] Teo PY, Yang C, Whilding LM, *et al.* Ovarian cancer immunotherapy using PD-L1 siRNA targeted delivery from folic acid-functionalized polyethylenimine: strategies to enhance T cell killing. Adv Healthc Mater 2015; 4(8): 1180-9. [http://dx.doi.org/10.1002/adhm.201500089] [PMID: 25866054]

[44] Roeven MW, Hobo W, van der Voort R, Fredrix H, Norde WJ, Teijgeler K, *et al.* Efficient nontoxic delivery of PD-L1 and PD-L2 siRNA into dendritic cell vaccines using the cationic lipid SAINT-18. Journal of immunotherapy (Hagerstown, Md : 1997) 2015; 38(4): 145-54. [PMID: 25839440]

[45] Xu Z, Wang Y, Zhang L, Huang L. Nanoparticle-delivered transforming growth factor-β siRNA enhances vaccination against advanced melanoma by modifying tumor microenvironment. ACS Nano 2014; 8(4): 3636-45. [http://dx.doi.org/10.1021/nn500216y] [PMID: 24580381]

[46] Christian DA, Hunter CA. Particle-mediated delivery of cytokines for immunotherapy. Immunotherapy 2012; 4(4): 425-41. [http://dx.doi.org/10.2217/imt.12.26] [PMID: 22512636]

[47] Kedar E, Braun E, Rutkowski Y, Emanuel N, Barenholz Y. Delivery of cytokines by liposomes. II. Interleukin-2 encapsulated in long-circulating sterically stabilized liposomes: immunomodulatory and anti-tumor activity in mice. J Immunotherapy with emphasis on tumor immunology: Official J Soc for Biological Therapy 1994; 16(2): 115-24. [PMID: 7804526]

[48] ten Hagen TL, Seynhaeve AL, van Tiel ST, Ruiter DJ, Eggermont AM. Pegylated liposomal tumor necrosis factor-alpha results in reduced toxicity and synergistic antitumor activity after systemic administration in combination with liposomal doxorubicin (Doxil) in soft tissue sarcoma-bearing rats. Int J Cancer 2002; 97(1): 115-20. [http://dx.doi.org/10.1002/ijc.1578] [PMID: 11774252]

[49] Neelapu SS, Gause BL, Harvey L, Lee S-T, Frye AR, Horton J, *et al.* A novel proteoliposomal vaccine induces antitumor immunity against follicular lymphoma. Blood. 2007; 109(12): 5160-3. [http://dx.doi.org/10.1182/blood-2006-12-063594] [PMID: 17339422]

[50] Anderson PM, Hanson DC, Hasz DE, Halet MR, Blazar BR, Ochoa AC. Cytokines in liposomes: Preliminary studies with IL-1, IL-2, IL-6, GM-CSF and interferon-γ. Cytokine 1994; 6(1): 92-101.

[51] Stephan MT, Moon JJ, Um SH, Bershteyn A, Irvine DJ. Therapeutic cell engineering with surface-conjugated synthetic nanoparticles. Nat Med 2010; 16(9): 1035-41. [http://dx.doi.org/10.1038/nm.2198] [PMID: 20711198]

[52] Ahmed KK, Geary SM, Salem AK. Surface engineering tumor cells with adjuvant-loaded particles for use as cancer vaccines. J Control Release Soc 2017; 248: 1-9. [http://dx.doi.org/10.1016/j.jconrel.2016.12.036] [PMID: 28057523]

[53] Yuan H, Jiang W, von Roemeling CA, Qie Y, Liu X, Chen Y, *et al.* Multivalent bi-specific nanobioconjugate engager for targeted cancer immunotherapy. Nature Nanotechn 2017; 12(8): 763-9.

[http://dx.doi.org/10.1038/nnano.2017.69]

[54] Topalian Suzanne L, Drake Charles G, Pardoll Drew M. Immune checkpoint blockade: a common denominator approach to cancer therapy. Cancer Cell 2015; 27(4): 450-61. [http://dx.doi.org/10.1016/j.ccell.2015.03.001]

[55] Leach DR, Krummel MF, Allison JP. Enhancement of antitumor immunity by CTLA-4 blockade. Science 1996; 271(5256): 1734-6. [http://dx.doi.org/10.1126/science.271.5256.1734] [PMID: 8596936]

[56] Freeman GJ, Long AJ, Iwai Y, *et al.* Engagement of the PD-1 immunoinhibitory receptor by a novel B7 family member leads to negative regulation of lymphocyte activation. J Exp Med 2000; 192(7): 1027-34. [http://dx.doi.org/10.1084/jem.192.7.1027] [PMID: 11015443]

[57] Pardoll DM. The blockade of immune checkpoints in cancer immunotherapy. Nat Rev Cancer 2012; 12(4): 252-64. [http://dx.doi.org/10.1038/nrc3239] [PMID: 22437870]

[58] Arlauckas SP, Garris CS, Kohler RH, *et al.* In vivo imaging reveals a tumor-associated macrophage-mediated resistance pathway in anti-PD-1 therapy. Sci Transl Med 2017; 9(389): eaal3604. [http://dx.doi.org/10.1126/scitranslmed.aal3604] [PMID: 28490665]

[59] Li S-Y, Liu Y, Xu C-F, *et al.* Restoring anti-tumor functions of T cells *via* nanoparticle-mediated immune checkpoint modulation. J Control Release 2016; 231: 17-28. [http://dx.doi.org/10.1016/j.jconrel.2016.01.044] [PMID: 26829099]

[60] Patel SP, Kurzrock R. PD-L1 expression as a predictive biomarker in cancer immunotherapy. Mol Cancer Ther 2015; 14(4): 847-56. [http://dx.doi.org/10.1158/1535-7163.MCT-14-0983] [PMID: 25695955]

[61] Spranger S, Spaapen RM, Zha Y, Williams J, Meng Y, Ha TT, *et al.* Up-regulation of PD-L1, IDO, and T(regs) in the melanoma tumor microenvironment is driven by CD8(+) T cells. Science translational medicine 2013; 5(200): 200ra116-200ra116. [PMID: 23986400]

[62] Kluger HM, Zito CR, Barr ML, Baine MK, Chiang VL, Sznol M, *et al.* Characterization of PD-L1 expression and associated t-cell infiltrates in metastatic melanoma samples from variable anatomic sites. Clin Cancer Res 2015; 21(13): 3052-60. [PMID: 25788491]

[63] Hamanishi J, Mandai M, Iwasaki M, Okazaki T, Tanaka Y, Yamaguchi K, *et al.* Programmed cell death 1 ligand 1 and tumor-infiltrating CD8+ T lymphocytes are prognostic factors of human ovarian cancer. Proc Natl Acad Sci USA 2007; 104(9): 3360-5. [PMID: 17360651]

[64] Reck M, Rodríguez-Abreu D, Robinson AG, *et al.* KEYNOTE-024 Investigators. Pembrolizumab *versus* chemotherapy for PD-L1-positive non-small-cell lung cancer. N Engl J Med 2016; 375(19): 1823-33. [http://dx.doi.org/10.1056/NEJMoa1606774] [PMID: 27718847]

[65] Müller T, Braun M, Dietrich D, *et al.* PD-L1: a novel prognostic biomarker in head and neck squamous cell carcinoma. Oncotarget 2017; 8(32): 52889-900. [http://dx.doi.org/10.18632/oncotarget.17547] [PMID: 28881780]

[66] Padda SK, Riess JW, Schwartz EJ, Tian L, Kohrt HE, Neal JW, *et al.* Diffuse high intensity PD-L1 staining in thymic epithelial tumors. J Thoracic 2015; 10(3): 500-8. [PMID: 25402569]

[67] Kiyasu J, Miyoshi H, Hirata A, *et al.* Expression of programmed cell death ligand 1 is associated with

poor overall survival in patients with diffuse large B-cell lymphoma. Blood 2015; 126(19): 2193-201. [http://dx.doi.org/10.1182/blood-2015-02-629600] [PMID: 26239088]

[68] Wang C, Sun W, Ye Y, Hu Q, Bomba H, Gu Z. *In situ* activation of platelets with checkpoint inhibitors for post-surgical cancer immunotherapy. Nature Biomedical Engineering 2017; 1: 0011. [http://dx.doi.org/10.1038/s41551-016-0011]

[69] McHugh MD, Park J, Uhrich R, Gao W, Horwitz DA, Fahmy TM. Paracrine co-delivery of TGF-β and IL-2 using CD4-targeted nanoparticles for induction and maintenance of regulatory T cells. Biomaterials 2015; 59: 172-81. [http://dx.doi.org/10.1016/j.biomaterials.2015.04.003] [PMID: 25974747]

[70] Stephan MT, Stephan SB, Bak P, Chen J, Irvine DJ. Synapse-directed delivery of immunomodulators using T-cell-conjugated nanoparticles. Biomaterials 2012; 33(23): 5776-87. [http://dx.doi.org/10.1016/j.biomaterials.2012.04.029] [PMID: 22594972]

[71] Schmid D, Park CG, Hartl CA, *et al.* T cell-targeting nanoparticles focus delivery of immunotherapy to improve antitumor immunity. Nat Commun 2017; 8(1): 1747. [http://dx.doi.org/10.1038/s41467-017-01830-8] [PMID: 29170511]

[72] Wang C, Ye Y, Hochu GM, Sadeghifar H, Gu Z. Enhanced cancer immunotherapy by microneedle patch-assisted delivery of Anti-PD1 antibody. Nano Letters 2016; 16(4): 2334-40. [http://dx.doi.org/10.1021/acs.nanolett.5b05030]

[73] Ye Y, Wang J, Hu Q, *et al.* Synergistic transcutaneous immunotherapy enhances antitumor immune responses through delivery of checkpoint inhibitors. ACS Nano 2016; 10(9): 8956-63. [http://dx.doi.org/10.1021/acsnano.6b04989] [PMID: 27599066]

[74] Krysko DV, Garg AD, Kaczmarek A, Krysko O, Agostinis P, Vandenabeele P. Immunogenic cell death and DAMPs in cancer therapy. Nat Rev Cancer 2012; 12(12): 860-75. [http://dx.doi.org/10.1038/nrc3380] [PMID: 23151605]

[75] Golden EB, Frances D, Pellicciotta I, Demaria S, Helen Barcellos-Hoff M, Formenti SC. Radiation fosters dose-dependent and chemotherapy-induced immunogenic cell death. OncoImmunology 2014; 3: e28518. [http://dx.doi.org/10.4161/onci.28518] [PMID: 25071979]

[76] Tanaka M, Kataoka H, Yano S, *et al.* Immunogenic cell death due to a new photodynamic therapy (PDT) with glycoconjugated chlorin (G-chlorin). Oncotarget 2016; 7(30): 47242-51. [http://dx.doi.org/10.18632/oncotarget.9725] [PMID: 27363018]

[77] Zhou F, Wu S, Song S, Chen WR, Resasco DE, Xing D. Antitumor immunologically modified carbon nanotubes for photothermal therapy. Biomaterials 2012; 33(11): 3235-42. [http://dx.doi.org/10.1016/j.biomaterials.2011.12.029] [PMID: 22296829]

[78] Kono K, Mimura K, Kiessling R. Immunogenic tumor cell death induced by chemoradiotherapy: molecular mechanisms and a clinical translation. Cell Death Dis 2013; 4(6): e688-e. [http://dx.doi.org/10.1038/cddis.2013.207] [PMID: 23788045]

[79] Obeid M, Tesniere A, Ghiringhelli F, *et al.* Calreticulin exposure dictates the immunogenicity of cancer cell death. Nat Med 2007; 13(1): 54-61. [http://dx.doi.org/10.1038/nm1523] [PMID: 17187072]

[80] Pfirschke C, Engblom C, Rickelt S, *et al.* Immunogenic chemotherapy sensitizes tumors to checkpoint blockade therapy. Immunity 2016; 44(2): 343-54. [http://dx.doi.org/10.1016/j.immuni.2015.11.024] [PMID: 26872698]

[81] van der Sluis TC, van Duikeren S, Huppelschoten S, Jordanova ES, Beyranvand Nejad E, Sloots A, *et al.* Vaccine-induced tumor necrosis factor-producing T cells synergize with cisplatin to promote tumor cell death. Clin Cancer Res 2015; 21(4): 781-94. [http://dx.doi.org/10.1158/1078-0432.CCR-14-2142] [PMID: 25501579]

[82] Alizadeh D, Trad M, Hanke NT, *et al.* Doxorubicin eliminates myeloid-derived suppressor cells and enhances the efficacy of adoptive T-cell transfer in breast cancer. Cancer Res 2014; 74(1): 104-18. [http://dx.doi.org/10.1158/0008-5472.CAN-13-1545] [PMID: 24197130]

[83] Zhang Z, Yu X, Wang Z, Wu P, Huang J. Anthracyclines potentiate anti-tumor immunity: A new opportunity for chemoimmunotherapy. Cancer Lett 2015; 369(2): 331-5. [http://dx.doi.org/10.1016/j.canlet.2015.10.002] [PMID: 26454214]

[84] Makkouk A, Joshi VB, Wongrakpanich A, *et al.* Biodegradable microparticles loaded with doxorubicin and CpG ODN for in situ immunization against cancer. AAPS J 2015; 17(1): 184-93. [http://dx.doi.org/10.1208/s12248-014-9676-6] [PMID: 25331103]

[85] Zhao X, Yang K, Zhao R, *et al.* Inducing enhanced immunogenic cell death with nanocarrier-based drug delivery systems for pancreatic cancer therapy. Biomaterials 2016; 102: 187-97. [http://dx.doi.org/10.1016/j.biomaterials.2016.06.032] [PMID: 27343466]

[86] Guo L, Yan DD, Yang D, Li Y, Wang X, Zalewski O, *et al.* Combinatorial photothermal and immuno cancer therapy using chitosan-coated hollow copper sulfide nanoparticles. ACS Nano 2014; 8(6): 5670-81.
[http://dx.doi.org/10.1021/nn5002112]

[87] Dreaden EC, Austin LA, Mackey MA, El-Sayed MA. Size matters: gold nanoparticles in targeted cancer drug delivery. Ther Deliv 2012; 3(4): 457-78. [http://dx.doi.org/10.4155/tde.12.21] [PMID: 22834077]

[88] Curnis F, Fiocchi M, Sacchi A, Gori A, Gasparri A, Corti A. NGR-tagged nano-gold: A new CD13-selective carrier for cytokine delivery to tumors. Nano Res 2016; 9(5): 1393-408. [http://dx.doi.org/10.1007/s12274-016-1035-8] [PMID: 27226823]

[89] Meir R, Shamalov K, Sadan T, Motiei M, Yaari G, Cohen CJ, *et al.* Fast image-guided stratification using anti-programmed death ligand 1 gold nanoparticles for cancer immunotherapy. ACS Nano 2017; 11(11): 11127-34.

[90] Wang X, Li X, Ito A, *et al.* Biodegradable metal ion-doped mesoporous silica nanospheres stimulate anticancer Th1 immune response *in vivo* . ACS Appl Mater Interfaces 2017; 9(50): 43538-44. [http://dx.doi.org/10.1021/acsami.7b16118] [PMID: 29192493]

[91] An M, Li M, Xi J, Liu H. Silica nanoparticle as a Lymph node targeting platform for vaccine delivery. ACS Appl Mater Interfaces 2017; 9(28): 23466-75. [http://dx.doi.org/10.1021/acsami.7b06024] [PMID: 28640587]

[92] Lu J, Liu X, Liao YP, Salazar F, Sun B, Jiang W, *et al.* Nano-enabled pancreas cancer immunotherapy using immunogenic cell death and reversing immunosuppression. Nat Commun 2017; 8(1): 1811. [http://dx.doi.org/10.1038/s41467-017-01651-9] [PMID: 29180759]

[93] Kienzle A, Kurch S, Schlöder J, *et al.* Dendritic Mesoporous Silica Nanoparticles for pH-Stimul--Responsive Drug Delivery of TNF-Alpha. Adv Healthc Mater 2017; 6(13) [http://dx.doi.org/10.1002/adhm.201700012] [PMID: 28557249]

[94] Lu Y, Yang Y, Gu Z, Zhang J, Song H, Xiang G, *et al.* Glutathione-depletion mesoporous organosilica nanoparticles as a self-adjuvant and Co-delivery platform for enhanced cancer immunotherapy. Biomat 2018; 175: 82-92.
[http://dx.doi.org/10.1016/j.biomaterials.2018.05.025]

[95] Lu J, Liu X, Liao YP, *et al.* Breast Cancer Chemo-immunotherapy through Liposomal Delivery of an Immunogenic Cell Death Stimulus Plus Interference in the IDO-1 Pathway. ACS Nano 2018; 12(11): 11041-61.
[http://dx.doi.org/10.1021/acsnano.8b05189] [PMID: 30481959]

[96] Meraz IM, Savage DJ, Segura-Ibarra V, Li J, Rhudy J, Gu J, *et al.* Adjuvant cationic liposomes presenting MPL and IL-12 induce cell death, suppress tumor growth, and alter the cellular phenotype of tumors in a murine model of breast cancer. Molecular Pharmaceutics 2014; 11(10): 3484-91.

[PMID: 25179345]

[97] Zhang Y, Li N, Suh H, Irvine DJ. Nanoparticle anchoring targets immune agonists to tumors enabling anti-cancer immunity without systemic toxicity. Nat Commun 2018 Jan 2; 9(1):6. [http://dx.doi.org/10.1038/s41467-017-02251-3] [PMID: 29295974]

[98] Chen Q, Xu L, Liang C, Wang C, Peng R, Liu Z. Photothermal therapy with immune-adjuvant nanoparticles together with checkpoint blockade for effective cancer immunotherapy. Nat Commun 2016; 7: 13193. [http://dx.doi.org/10.1038/ncomms13193] [PMID: 27767031]

[99] Sato-Kaneko F, Yao S, Ahmadi A, *et al.* Combination immunotherapy with TLR agonists and checkpoint inhibitors suppresses head and neck cancer. JCI Insight 2017; 2(18): 93397. [http://dx.doi.org/10.1172/jci.insight.93397] [PMID: 28931759]

[100] Nuhn L, De Koker S, Van Lint S, Zhong Z, Catani JP, Combes F, *et al.* Nanoparticle-conjugate TLR7/8 agonist localized immunotherapy provokes safe antitumoral responses. Advanced Materials (Deerfield Beach, Fla). 2018; 30(45): e1803397. [PMID: 30276880]

[101] Chen WL, Liu SJ, Leng CH, Chen HW, Chong P, Huang MH. Disintegration and cancer immunotherapy efficacy of a squalane-in-water delivery system emulsified by bioresorbable poly(ethylene glycol)-block-polylactide. Biomaterials 2014; 35(5): 1686-95. [http://dx.doi.org/10.1016/j.biomaterials.2013.11.004] [PMID: 24268203]

[102] Broaders KE, Cohen JA, Beaudette TT, Bachelder EM, Fréchet JMJ. Acetalated dextran is a chemically and biologically tunable material for particulate immunotherapy. Proc Natl Acad Sci USA 2009; 106(14): 5497-502. [http://dx.doi.org/10.1073/pnas.0901592106] [PMID: 19321415]

[103] Watkins-Schulz R, Tiet P, Gallovic MD, *et al.* A microparticle platform for STING-targeted immunotherapy enhances natural killer cell- and $CD8^+$ T cell-mediated anti-tumor immunity. Biomaterials 2019; 205: 94-105. [http://dx.doi.org/10.1016/j.biomaterials.2019.03.011] [PMID: 30909112]

[104] Peine KJ, Bachelder EM, Vangundy Z, Papenfuss T, Brackman DJ, Gallovic MD, *et al.* Efficient delivery of the toll-like receptor agonists polyinosinic:polycytidylic acid and CpG to macrophages by acetalated dextran microparticles. Molecular Pharma 2013; 10(8): 2849-57.

CHAPTER 10

Nanoparticle Vaccines

Abstract: As a result of new emerging pathological conditions, new microorganisms have set a challenge in front of the researchers for the development of treatment and vaccination strategies. In the area of vaccine development, new effects have been made to invent new vaccines and also to improve the efficacy of the currently available vaccines. A wide variety of vaccines have been developed from killed whole organisms, subunits and RNA or DNA fractions. To overcome the side effects of these vaccines, nanoparticles may carry the payload and deliver them on the target site. The nanoparticles have the potential to improve the efficacy of these antigens and reduce the side effects to a large extent . These nanoparticles should have the ability of safe delivery of the antigens, protect them from degradation, control release and biocompatible. In this study, we intended to discuss different characteristics of the nanoparticles along with their properties and the variety of payloads for immunstimulation.

Keywords: AIDS, Calcium phosphate, Carbon nanoparticle, Chitosan nanoparticle, Cytokines, DNA, Gold nanoparticle, Hydrophobicity, Immunstimulator, Inorganic nanoconjugate, Liposomal nanoparticle, Nanotechnology, Nucleic acid, Organic nanoconjugate, Polymeric nanoconjugate, RNA, Silica nanoparticle, Surface charge, Surface modification, Toll like receptors, Tuberculosis.

INTRODUCTION

In this century, the infectious diseases have emerged as a new threat to the mankind. Many new diseases have been reported and several old disease conditions have re-emerged that were considered to be no longer a threat for the human being [1 - 3]. Collectively, these disease conditions all together have an enormous adverse impact on the socioeconomic condition and health care sector. The major challenge of these new disease conditions is that they do not have any effective drug for the treatment of them.

In this era of nanotechnology, there are possibilities of development of new nanoparticles that may conjugate with a wide variety of payloads and may be used for the treatment of these presently incurable disease conditions [4]. These

Rituparna Acharya

incurable diseases include acquired immune deficiency syndrome (AIDS) and tuberculosis. The current need of the hour is to develop vaccines for these diseases. While developing vaccines, the main points that need to be kept in mind are the stability, safety and the ability to develop durable and adequate immune response in minimum dosage [5 - 7]. Currently, the available first generation, second generation and third generation vaccines are nothing but the attenuated or whole killed organism, subunit and RNA or DNA vaccines respectively [8 - 10]. However, there are several challenges in the delivery of these vaccines to the target site. To overcome these hurdles, nanoparticles may carry these vaccines to the target site with minimal side effects and dosage. They have the ability to protect the molecule from degradation, have good adjuvant property and deliver to the antigen presenting cell as a target. The nanoparticles may carry the molecule encapsulated within them that will protect them from degradation or they may be adsorbed on to the surface that may help them to interact with the tool like receptor on the surface of antigen presenting cells [11]. Nanoparticle based delivery of the antigens is a suitable route of administration as they help in cellular uptake and lead to a robust innate, humoral and cellular immunity.

In this study, we intended to describe the characteristics of the wide variety of nanocarriers, their different types and the immunostimulators *i.e.*, the payload of these nanocarriers.

CHARACTERIZATION OF NANOVACCINES

In order to enhance delivery and characteristics of vaccination, vaccine molecules are conjugated with the nanocarriers. Nanocarriers may provide surface conjugation [12] or encapsulation [13, 14] or surface adsorption [15, 16] of the vaccine molecule. However, the nano-immuno formulation provides improved antigen delivery and presentation to the immune system of our body [17]. In this regard, the size, shape, surface specificity *etc.* are the main key factors that affect the circulation, bioavailability, biodistribution and specificity of the nanoconjugate [18, 19]. Here, in this study, the physiochemical properties such as size, surface charge, shape, hydrophobicity, surface modification, *etc.* of the nanoconjugate are discussed.

Size

The size of the nanoparticles largely determines the cellular uptake of the nanoconjugate by the dendritic cells and antigen presenting cells [20, 21]. Large nanoparticles have reduced cellular internalization rate than smaller nanoparticles [22]. Smaller nanoparticles with a 20-200nm range are readily internalized by resident dendritic cells; on the other hand, larger nanoparticles that have a range between 500-2,000nm are effectively taken up by migratory dendritic cells [23].

Nanoparticles smaller than 200nm are drained by lymphatic system [24], while 20nm sized nanoparticles are transported to antigen presenting cells [25]. Notably, the cellular interaction and phagocytic rate of the nanoconjugate are also largely affected by the curvature of the nanoparticle [26]. Moreover, in cell signaling process, smaller nanoparticles have greater efficacy than larger one [27].

Surface Charge

Surface charge of the nanoparticle largely affects the specificity of the target site of the nanoconjugate. The surface charge interacts with the surface molecules present on the target cells. For example, cationic surface charged nanoparticle are efficiently internalized by the antigen presenting cells in comparison with the nanoparticle that have a neutral surface charge. This is because of the electrostatic interaction between the negatively charges cell membrane and positively charged nanoparticle [28, 29]. More examples of higher efficacy of positively surface charged nanoparticles are evidenced in several publications [30, 31]. Against infections, cationic nanoparticles are evidenced to be more effective than other forms in creating immunological reactions.

Shape

Other than size and surface charge, shapes of the nanoconjugates are the critical factor for cellular internalization, trafficking and antigen release within the host cells [32]. It has been demonstrated that spherical nanoparticles are more easily internalized by the cell and produce strong immune response than cubical or rod shaped nanoparticles [33 - 35]. Moreover, it is stated in a publication that although nanorods and nanosheets are internalized by the cell by clathrin-mediated endocytosis, nano rods are particularly delivered to the nucleus and nano sheets stay in the cytoplasm [36, 37]. It has been studied that enhanced antigen presentation and processing may be achieved only when the molecules are delivered in to the lysosomal compartment of the cell.

Hydrophobicity

Through the recognition of hydrophobic moieties, the nanoparticles have a critical role in the interaction of immune cells and soluble proteins [38]. Several publications have demonstrated that hydrophobic molecules have the property to induce cytokines and co-stimulatory molecules better than hydrophilic nanoparticles [39 - 41]. Enhanced activation of dendritic cells and innate immune cells was demonstrated in some publications by the hydrophobic nanoparticles in a highly potent form that in turn enhances the opsonization process by the absorption of immunoglobulin on the cell surface in an increased level [42, 43]. However, PEGylation inhibits the interaction of the nanoparticle with the immune cells that ultimately reduces their uptake by antigen presenting cells. Moreover, the incorporation of an alkyl linker between the thiol moieties and PEG on NPs may have the same effect as previously mentioned [44, 45].

Surface Modification

Nanoparticles may be surface modified that have several effects such as they alter the ligand specificity and their interaction with antigen presenting cells [25]. Nanoparticles may be conjugated with CD47 molecules that have effect of downstream signaling cascade and they are not internalized by phagocytic cells [46]. Up-regulation of cytokine production and immune regulatory genes may be achieved by functionalization of the nanoparticle with several Tool-Like Receptors such as TLR7, TLR-8 and TLR-9 agonists [47 - 49]. Activation of complement pathway may also be achieved by conjugation of the nanoparticles by several variety of molecules was published in several papers [14, 15]. Overall, from these publications, this may be concluded that by conjugation of molecules with nanoparticles and changing their physiochemical properties may help in delivering the vaccine molecule in specific site and enhancing the immune response.

NANOPARTICLE VACCINES

Nanoparticles are the most used nanomaterials in vaccine delivery. The nanoconjugates comprise three main components such as nanoparticle; immunogens or immune modulatory agents; and targeting ligands. Among these agents, nanoparticles have special property of cellular internalization, trafficking and also biodegradability and biocompatibility. The immunogens that are the main important part of the nanoconjugate may bind with the nanoparticle by adsorption on the surface or by conjugation or by encapsulation. Moreover, ligand incorporation with these nanoconjugates helps to elicited inflammatory responses and activates receptors on the surface of various immune cells.

The physiochemical characteristics of nanoparticles largely affect its vaccine efficacy and cellular uptake mechanism [50]. 20-200nm size nanoparticles are mainly ingested by dendritic cells by endocytosis. Larger particle s with size between .5-5μm are taken up by macropinocytosis and particles greater than 5μm are taken up by macrophages by phagocytosis method [51, 52].

On the other hand size of the nanoconjugates also has critical property on activation of immune cells. For example 40-50nm nano conjugates may promote the Type 1 T-cell response, whereas larger particles that have size larger than 500nm may activate Type 2 T-cell response and antibody activation [28].

Nanoparticles may be of different types such as inorganic, organic and polymeric nanoparticles. In this section we are intended to discuss about various forms of nanoconjugates that may be used for the vaccination method.

Inorganic Nanoconjugates

Gold, carbon, silica, calcium phosphate are the types of inorganic nanoparticles that are exploited in the delivery of vaccine [32, 44, 45, 53 - 55]. These nanoparticles may be fabricated in tailor made formats with wide variety of size, shapes and surface modifications. Various viral antigens are delivered through nanoparticle that helps to protect them from enzymatic degradation and prolong the antigen stability. In several disease conditions such as influenza, foot and mouth, immunodeficiency virus, andtuberculosis diseases in mice, the specific viral or bacterial antigens are delivered through gold nanoparticle leads to induction of robust host immune responses [56 - 59]. Plasmid DNA encoding bacterial antigen encapsulated within gold nanoparticle demonstrated high efficacy in reduction of burden of infection in mice [57, 58]. Along with the DNA vaccines gold nanoparticles may also deliver protein [12, 60], peptide [44] and conjugate vaccines [61]. Other nanoparticles such as mesosporous silica, a spherical form of carbon nanoparticle and nanotube also helps in the delivery of protein and peptide antigens that improves immunogenicity against viral infection [32, 59, 62]. Silica nanoparticles also have advantages as they have abundant silanol groups on their surface that makes them accessible of the vaccine molecules to the target site [62 - 64]. Moreover, albumin loaded silica nanoparticles are able to induce humoral and cellular immunity [65]. Magnetic nanoparticles are another type of inorganic nanoparticle that helps in vaccine delivery [66 - 68]. Inorganic nanoparticles have advantages as they are biocompatible, they have low production cost and reproducibility.

Organic Nanoconjugates

Other than inorganic nanoparticles organic nanoparticles are also widely explored area of research in vaccine delivery. Liposomes are the most widely used organic nanoparticle in delivery of wide variety of payloads. It has been reported that T-cell and B-cell response may be elicited by the delivery of antigenic protein entrapped multilamellar lipid vesicles [42]. Similarly, phosphatidylserine (PS)-liposomes conjugated with antigenic peptides may potentiate T-helper cell response and leads to the internalization of the nanoconjugate by antigen presenting cells [43]. Strong protective immunity was also elicited against fungal infection by liposomal nanoconjugate that delivers heat shock protein encoding vaccine DNA [69]. Several liposomal nanoparticle based vaccines are in clinical trial against wide variety of disease conditions [40]. One of such study demonstrated that liposomal aerosol carrier is potent generator of immunity against tuberculosis [70, 71]. Other studies also shown that influenza, chlamydia, tuberculosis, and erythrocytic-stage malaria infections may be protected by dimethyl dioctadecyl ammonium (DDA) lipid based liposomes [72 - 76]. The DNA vaccine in conjugation with liposomes is also delivered in the lung of the monkey successfully [77].

Polymeric Nanoconjugates

Polymeric nanoconjugates are being used in broad range of disease conditions with wide variety of antigens in conjugation including hepatitis-B virus antigens [78], hydrophobicantigens [34, 79], *Bacillus anthracis* [80], ovalbumin [81], and tetanus toxoid [79]. PLGA-antigen nanoconjugate demonstrated the property of eliciting immunostimulation against mycobacteria infection by inducing cytokines and nitric oxide production [82]. Along with the synthetic polymers, some natural polymers are also used as adjuvants for example alginate, inulins, pullans and chitosan [83 - 86]. Inulins are the protector of influenza virus and hepatitis B by activating complement system [87]. Similarly, chitosan nanoparticle may be conjugated with Newcastle disease vaccine [88], HBV antigens [89] and DNA vaccine [90]. The delivery of vaccines is more potent at the mucosal site by chitosan and PLGA nanoparticle delivery [91, 92]. The intradermal and intra peritoneal administration of nanoconjugates are highly discussed in today's research [93]. Many such nanoconjugates are in preclinical stage as they are already known for the biocompatibility and reduced toxicity *in vitro* and *in vivo* conditions [94].

IMMUNE STIMULATOR USING NANOCARRIER

Cytokines

Cytokines are the signaling molecules that are secreted by wide variety of cells in response to immunological reactions. Among other activities cytokines have an ability to activate different immune cells to protect our body from different disease conditions. However, these cytokines have certain drawbacks as they are susceptible to early degradation as uncontrolled release of these substances may lead to harmful effects [30]. In this regards, to overcome these problems wide variety of nanocarriers are designed to deliver the above said particles to the target site. This remedial approach have decreased their cytotoxic effect, improved the half-life and activation of T-cells in response to the cytokines [95, 96]. This principle is also applicable for cancer therapy by incorporating interferon alpha

(IFN-a)and granulocyte macrophage colonystimulating factor (GM-CSF) within the nanocarrier [31, 97]. Moreover, in case of infectious diseases this method may be applied by incorporating IL-12 in microspheres to protect against tuberculosis. The sustained release of this IL-12 from the nanoconjugate helps in the production of antibodies in higher concentration [98].

Toll Like Receptor Agonists

In research several Toll Like Receptor agonists are explored as an immune activator. Wide variety of Toll Like Receptors are expressed in immune cells such as macrophages, B-cells and dendritic cells that interacts with specific pathogen associatedmolecular patterns (PAMPs). This ligand-receptor interaction activates several downstream signaling cascades that eliminates or generates immune response against pathogens [46, 47]. Several publications have documented that Toll Like Receptor agonist in conjugation with nanoparticles have prolonged and enhanced T-cell response [48, 49, 99] and helped in activation and maturation of the dendritic cells [93]. These publications have explored the possibility of the application of these nanoconjugates in targeting the lymph organs rich with T-cells and B-cells.

Nucleic Acids

Nucleic acids are considered to be the next generation vaccines as they may act as an immuno-stimulant. Plasmids may be used to translocate to the nucleus and transcribe fusion antigens that may act as an immune-stimulant [100]. Similarly, many such studies have been conducted on DNA and RNA molecules that may produce antigens and capable of generating humoral and cellular immune responses [101]. Likewise, plasmids comprising of viral antigen encoding genes may be encapsulated in a nanocarrier may be used to target viral infection [102].

CONCLUSION

The nano-immuno formulations have several advantages such as they have improved antigen stability, enhanced immunogenicity properties and targeted delivery ability. Largely, the soluble antigens are poor inducer of protective immunity and inefficiently endocytosed by antigen presenting cells. However, the recognition and uptake of these soluble antigens by antigen presenting cells may be improved by conjugating them with nanocarriers. This strategy is applicable for polysaccharides of pneumococcal vaccines that help to improve the immunogenicity of the poorly immunogenic antigens [103]. Recently, with the development of nanotechnology, a wide variety of nano-vaccines is growing with their new strategies of synthesis methods. Moreover, the growth of new nano formulations in conjugation with immunostimulatory substances enhanced the adjuvant property of the nanoparticles and subsequent cellular activation. Nanoparticles may be tailor-made for their long-time delivery in a single-dose in a specific location. Multiple studies have demonstrated the possibility of non-invasive administration of vaccines in multiple locations [104 - 109]. Thus, the progress of research may develop a nanoconjugate that not only has immunogenic property but also has the ability to combat infection.

REFERENCES

[1] Kahn RE, Ma W, Richt JA. Swine and influenza: a challenge to one health research. Curr Top Microbiol Immunol 2014; 385: 205-18.
[http://dx.doi.org/10.1007/82_2014_392] [PMID: 25005926]

[2] Braden CR, Dowell SF, Jernigan DB, Hughes JM. Progress in global surveillance and response capacity 10 years after severe acute respiratory syndrome. Emerg Infect Dis 2013; 19(6): 864-9.
[http://dx.doi.org/10.3201/eid1906.130192] [PMID: 23731871]

[3] Wejse C, Patsche CB, Kühle A, Bamba FJV, Mendes MS, Lemvik G, *et al.* Impact of HIV-1, HIV-2, and HIV-1+2 dual infection on the outcome of tuberculosis. Intern J Infectious Dis 2015; 32: 128-34.

[4] Greenwood B. The contribution of vaccination to global health: past, present and future. Philos Trans R Soc Lond B Biol Sci 2014; 369(1645): 20130433.
[http://dx.doi.org/10.1098/rstb.2013.0433] [PMID: 24821919]

[5] Ada GL. The ideal vaccine. World J Microbiol Biotechnol 1991; 7(2): 105-9.
[http://dx.doi.org/10.1007/BF00328978] [PMID: 24424920]

[6] Atkins HS, Morton M, Griffin KF, Stokes MG, Nataro JP, Titball RW. Recombinant salmonella vaccines for biodefence. Vaccine 2006; 24(15): 2710-7.
[http://dx.doi.org/10.1016/j.vaccine.2005.12.046] [PMID: 16434131]

[7] Beverley PCL. Immunology of vaccination. Br Med Bull 2002; 62(1): 15-28.
[http://dx.doi.org/10.1093/bmb/62.1.15] [PMID: 12176847]

[8] Ulmer JB, Donnelly JJ, Parker SE, *et al.* Heterologous protection against influenza by injection of DNA encoding a viral protein. Science 1993; 259(5102): 1745-9.
[http://dx.doi.org/10.1126/science.8456302] [PMID: 8456302]

[9] Scallan CD, Tingley DW, Lindbloom JD, Toomey JS, Tucker SN. An adenovirus-based vaccine with a double-stranded RNA adjuvant protects mice and ferrets against H5N1 avian influenza in oral delivery models. Clin Vaccine Immunol 2013; 20(1): 85-94.
[http://dx.doi.org/10.1128/CVI.00552-12] [PMID: 23155123]

[10] Altenburg AF, Kreijtz JH, de Vries RD, *et al.* Modified vaccinia virus ankara (MVA) as production platform for vaccines against influenza and other viral respiratory diseases. Viruses 2014; 6(7): 2735-61.
[http://dx.doi.org/10.3390/v6072735] [PMID: 25036462]

[11] Means T, Hayashi F, Smith K, Aderem A, Luster A. The toll-like receptor 5 stimulus bacterial flagellin induces maturation and chemokine production in human dendritic cells. J Immun (Baltimore, Md : 1950) 2003; 170: 5165-75.

[12] Gregory AE, Williamson ED, Prior JL, *et al.* Conjugation of Y. pestis F1-antigen to gold nanoparticles improves immunogenicity. Vaccine 2012; 30(48): 6777-82.
[http://dx.doi.org/10.1016/j.vaccine.2012.09.021] [PMID: 23000121]

[13] He Q, Mitchell AR, Johnson SL, Wagner-Bartak C, Morcol T, Bell SJ. Calcium phosphate nanoparticle adjuvant. Clin Diagn Lab Immunol 2000; 7(6): 899-903.
[http://dx.doi.org/10.1128/CDLI.7.6.899-903.2000] [PMID: 11063495]

[14] Oyewumi MO, Kumar A, Cui Z. Nano-microparticles as immune adjuvants: correlating particle sizes and the resultant immune responses. Expert Rev Vaccines 2010; 9(9): 1095-107. [http://dx.doi.org/10.1586/erv.10.89] [PMID: 20822351]

[15] Wendorf J, Singh M, Chesko J, *et al.* A practical approach to the use of nanoparticles for vaccine delivery. J Pharm Sci 2006; 95(12): 2738-50. [http://dx.doi.org/10.1002/jps.20728] [PMID: 16927245]

[16] Stieneker F, Kreuter J, Löwer J. High antibody titres in mice with polymethylmethacrylate nanoparticles as adjuvant for HIV vaccines. AIDS 1991; 5(4): 431-5. [http://dx.doi.org/10.1097/00002030-199104000-00012] [PMID: 2059385]

[17] Reddy ST, Rehor A, Schmoekel HG, Hubbell JA, Swartz MA. *In vivo* targeting of dendritic cells in lymph nodes with poly (propylene sulfide) nanoparticles. J. Control. Release Soc 2006; 112(1): 26-34. [PMID: 16529839]

[18] Sunshine JC, Perica K, Schneck JP, Green JJ. Particle shape dependence of CD8+ T cell activation by artificial antigen presenting cells. Biomaterials 2014; 35(1): 269-77. [http://dx.doi.org/10.1016/j.biomaterials.2013.09.050] [PMID: 24099710]

[19] Yameen B, Choi WI, Vilos C, Swami A, Shi J, Farokhzad OC. Insight into nanoparticle cellular uptake and intracellular targeting. J Controlled Rel 2014; 190: 485-99. [http://dx.doi.org/10.1016/j.jconrel.2014.06.038] [PMID: 24984011]

[20] Dobrovolskaia MA, Aggarwal P, Hall JB, McNeil SE. Preclinical studies to understand nanoparticle interaction with the immune system and its potential effects on nanoparticle biodistribution. Mol Pharm 2008; 5(4): 487-95. [http://dx.doi.org/10.1021/mp800032f] [PMID: 18510338]

[21] Zolnik BS, González-Fernández A, Sadrieh N, Dobrovolskaia MA. Nanoparticles and the immune system. Endocrinology 2010; 151(2): 458-65. [http://dx.doi.org/10.1210/en.2009-1082] [PMID: 20016026]

[22] Joshi VB, Geary SM, Salem AK. Biodegradable particles as vaccine delivery systems: size matters. AAPS J 2013; 15(1): 85-94. [http://dx.doi.org/10.1208/s12248-012-9418-6] [PMID: 23054976]

[23] Manolova V, Flace A, Bauer M, Schwarz K, Saudan P, Bachmann MF. Nanoparticles target distinct dendritic cell populations according to their size. Eur J Immunol 2008; 38(5): 1404-13. [http://dx.doi.org/10.1002/eji.200737984] [PMID: 18389478]

[24] Nishioka Y, Yoshino H. Lymphatic targeting with nanoparticulate system. Adv Drug Deliv Rev 2001; 47(1): 55-64. [http://dx.doi.org/10.1016/S0169-409X(00)00121-6] [PMID: 11251245]

[25] Reddy S, van der Vlies A, Simeoni E, Angeli V, Randolph G, O'Neil C, *et al.* Exploiting lymphatic transport and complement activation in nanoparticle vaccines. Nature Biotechn 2007; 25: 1159-64. [http://dx.doi.org/10.1038/nbt1332]

[26] Kostarelos K, Lacerda L, Pastorin G, *et al.* Cellular uptake of functionalized carbon nanotubes is independent of functional group and cell type. Nat Nanotechnol 2007; 2(2): 108-13. [http://dx.doi.org/10.1038/nnano.2006.209] [PMID: 18654229]

[27] Lim JS, Lee K, Choi JN, *et al.* Intracellular protein delivery by hollow mesoporous silica capsules with a large surface hole. Nanotechnology 2012; 23(8): 085101. [http://dx.doi.org/10.1088/0957-4484/23/8/085101] [PMID: 22293239]

[28] Foged C, Brodin B, Frokjaer S, Sundblad A. Particle size and surface charge affect particle uptake by human dendritic cells in an *in vitro* model. Int J Pharm 2005; 298(2): 315-22. [http://dx.doi.org/10.1016/j.ijpharm.2005.03.035] [PMID: 15961266]

[29] Thiele L, Merkle HP, Walter E. Phagocytosis and phagosomal fate of surface-modified microparticles in dendritic cells and macrophages. Pharm Res 2003; 20(2): 221-8. [http://dx.doi.org/10.1023/A:1022271020390] [PMID: 12636160]

[30] Jaffer U, Wade RG, Gourlay T. Cytokines in the systemic inflammatory response syndrome: a review. HSR Proc Intensive Care Cardiovasc Anesth 2010; 2(3): 161-75. [PMID: 23441054]

[31] Ali OA, Huebsch N, Cao L, Dranoff G, Mooney DJ. Infection-mimicking materials to program dendritic cells *in situ*. Nat Mater 2009; 8(2): 151-8. [http://dx.doi.org/10.1038/nmat2357] [PMID: 19136947]

[32] Wang T, Zou M, Jiang H, Ji Z, Gao P, Cheng G. Synthesis of a novel kind of carbon nanoparticle with large mesopores and macropores and its application as an oral vaccine adjuvant. Euro J Pharmaceu Sci: Official J European Federation for Pharmaceutical Sci 2011; 44(5): 653-9. [http://dx.doi.org/10.1016/j.ejps.2011.10.012] [PMID: 22064451]

[33] Prego C, Paolicelli P, Díaz B, *et al.* Chitosan-based nanoparticles for improving immunization against hepatitis B infection. Vaccine 2010; 28(14): 2607-14. [http://dx.doi.org/10.1016/j.vaccine.2010.01.011] [PMID: 20096389]

[34] Shen H, Ackerman AL, Cody V, *et al.* Enhanced and prolonged cross-presentation following endosomal escape of exogenous antigens encapsulated in biodegradable nanoparticles. Immunology 2006; 117(1): 78-88. [http://dx.doi.org/10.1111/j.1365-2567.2005.02268.x] [PMID: 16423043]

[35] Niikura K, Matsunaga T, Suzuki T, *et al.* Gold nanoparticles as a vaccine platform: influence of size and shape on immunological responses *in vitro* and *in vivo*. ACS Nano 2013; 7(5): 3926-38. [http://dx.doi.org/10.1021/nn3057005] [PMID: 23631767]

[36] Glück R, Moser C, Metcalfe IC. Influenza virosomes as an efficient system for adjuvanted vaccine delivery. Expert Opin Biol Ther 2004; 4(7): 1139-45. [http://dx.doi.org/10.1517/14712598.4.7.1139] [PMID: 15268680]

[37] Morein B, Sundquist B, Höglund S, Dalsgaard K, Osterhaus A. Iscom, a novel structure for antigenic presentation of membrane proteins from enveloped viruses. Nature 1984; 308(5958): 457-60. [http://dx.doi.org/10.1038/308457a0] [PMID: 6709052]

[38] Kim ST, Saha K, Kim C, Rotello VM. The role of surface functionality in determining nanoparticle cytotoxicity. Accounts of Chemical Res 2013; 46(3): 681-91. [http://dx.doi.org/10.1021/ar3000647]

[39] Raghuvanshi RS, Katare YK, Lalwani K, Ali MM, Singh O, Panda AK. Improved immune response from biodegradable polymer particles entrapping tetanus toxoid by use of different immunization protocol and adjuvants. Int J Pharm 2002; 245(1-2): 109-21. [http://dx.doi.org/10.1016/S0378-5173(02)00342-3] [PMID: 12270248]

[40] Watson DS, Endsley AN, Huang L. Design considerations for liposomal vaccines: influence of formulation parameters on antibody and cell-mediated immune responses to liposome associated antigens. Vaccine 2012; 30(13): 2256-72. [http://dx.doi.org/10.1016/j.vaccine.2012.01.070] [PMID: 22306376]

[41] Hillaireau H, Couvreur P. Nanocarriers' entry into the cell: relevance to drug delivery. Cell Mol Life Sci 2009; 66(17): 2873-96. [http://dx.doi.org/10.1007/s00018-009-0053-z] [PMID: 19499185]

[42] Moon JJ, Suh H, Bershteyn A, *et al.* Interbilayer-crosslinked multilamellar vesicles as synthetic vaccines for potent humoral and cellular immune responses. Nat Mater 2011; 10(3): 243-51. [http://dx.doi.org/10.1038/nmat2960] [PMID: 21336265]

[43] Ichihashi T, Satoh T, Sugimoto C, Kajino K. Emulsified phosphatidylserine, simple and effective peptide carrier for induction of potent epitope-specific T cell responses. PLoS One 2013; 8(3): e60068.

[http://dx.doi.org/10.1371/journal.pone.0060068] [PMID: 23533665]

[44] Chen YS, Hung YC, Lin WH, Huang GS. Assessment of gold nanoparticles as a size-dependent vaccine carrier for enhancing the antibody response against synthetic foot-and-mouth disease virus peptide. Nanotechnology 2010; 21(19): 195101. [http://dx.doi.org/10.1088/0957-4484/21/19/195101] [PMID: 20400818]

[45] Zhou X, Zhang X, Yu X, *et al.* The effect of conjugation to gold nanoparticles on the ability of low molecular weight chitosan to transfer DNA vaccine. Biomaterials 2008; 29(1): 111-7. [http://dx.doi.org/10.1016/j.biomaterials.2007.09.007] [PMID: 17905427]

[46] Kawai T, Akira S. Toll-like receptors and their crosstalk with other innate receptors in infection and immunity. Immunity 2011; 34(5): 637-50. [http://dx.doi.org/10.1016/j.immuni.2011.05.006] [PMID: 21616434]

[47] Schenten D, Medzhitov R. The control of adaptive immune responses by the innate immune system. Adv Immunol 2011; 109: 87-124. [http://dx.doi.org/10.1016/B978-0-12-387664-5.00003-0] [PMID: 21569913]

[48] Lynn GM, Laga R, Darrah PA, *et al.* In vivo characterization of the physicochemical properties of polymer-linked TLR agonists that enhance vaccine immunogenicity. Nat Biotechnol 2015; 33(11): 1201-10. [http://dx.doi.org/10.1038/nbt.3371] [PMID: 26501954]

[49] Goldinger SM, Dummer R, Baumgaertner P, Mihic-Probst D, Schwarz K, Hammann-Haenni A, *et al.* Nano-particle vaccination combined with TLR-7 and -9 ligands triggers memory and effector CD8□ T-cell responses in melanoma patients. Eur J Immun 2012; 42(11): 3049-61. [PMID: 22806397]

[50] Cu Y, Saltzman WM. Controlled surface modification with poly(ethylene)glycol enhances diffusion of PLGA nanoparticles in human cervical mucus. Mol Pharm 2009; 6(1): 173-81. [http://dx.doi.org/10.1021/mp8001254] [PMID: 19053536]

[51] Pelkmans L. Secrets of caveolae- and lipid raft-mediated endocytosis revealed by mammalian viruses. Biochim Biophys Acta 2005; 1746(3): 295-304. [http://dx.doi.org/10.1016/j.bbamcr.2005.06.009] [PMID: 16126288]

[52] Fifis T, Gamvrellis A, Crimeen-Irwin B, Pietersz GA, Li J, Mottram PL, *et al.* Size-dependent immunogenicity: therapeutic and protective properties of nano-vaccines against tumors. J Immun (Baltimore, Md: 1950). 2004; 173(5): 3148-54. [http://dx.doi.org/10.4049/jimmunol.173.5.3148] [PMID: 15322175]

[53] Turkevich J, Stevenson PC, Hillier J. A study of the nucleation and growth processes in the synthesis of colloidal gold. Discuss Faraday Soc 1951; 11(0): 55-75. [http://dx.doi.org/10.1039/df9511100055]

[54] He Q, Mitchell A, Morcol T, Bell SJD. Calcium phosphate nanoparticles induce mucosal immunity and protection against herpes simplex virus type 2. Clin Diagn Lab Immunol 2002; 9(5): 1021-4. [PMID: 12204953]

[55] Joyappa DH, Kumar CA, Banumathi N, Reddy GR, Suryanarayana VV. Calcium phosphate nanoparticle prepared with foot and mouth disease virus P1-3CD gene construct protects mice and guinea pigs against the challenge virus. Vet Microbiol 2009; 139(1-2): 58-66. [http://dx.doi.org/10.1016/j.vetmic.2009.05.004] [PMID: 19505774]

[56] Tao W, Gill HS. M2e-immobilized gold nanoparticles as influenza A vaccine: Role of soluble M2e and longevity of protection. Vaccine 2015; 33(20): 2307-15. [http://dx.doi.org/10.1016/j.vaccine.2015.03.063] [PMID: 25842219]

[57] Xu L, Liu Y, Chen Z, *et al.* Surface-engineered gold nanorods: promising DNA vaccine adjuvant for HIV-1 treatment. Nano Lett 2012; 12(4): 2003-12. [http://dx.doi.org/10.1021/nl300027p] [PMID: 22372996]

[58] Silva CL, Bonato VL, Coelho-Castelo AA, *et al.* Immunotherapy with plasmid DNA encoding mycobacterial hsp65 in association with chemotherapy is a more rapid and efficient form of treatment for tuberculosis in mice. Gene Ther 2005; 12(3): 281-7. [http://dx.doi.org/10.1038/sj.gt.3302418] [PMID: 15526006]

[59] Villa CH, Dao T, Ahearn I, *et al.* Single-walled carbon nanotubes deliver peptide antigen into dendritic cells and enhance IgG responses to tumor-associated antigens. ACS Nano 2011; 5(7): 5300-11. [http://dx.doi.org/10.1021/nn200182x] [PMID: 21682329]

[60] Tao W, Ziemer KS, Gill HS. Gold nanoparticle-M2e conjugate coformulated with CpG induces protective immunity against influenza A virus. Nanomedicine (Lond) 2014; 9(2): 237-51. [http://dx.doi.org/10.2217/nnm.13.58] [PMID: 23829488]

[61] Safari D, Marradi M, Chiodo F, *et al.* Gold nanoparticles as carriers for a synthetic Streptococcus pneumoniae type 14 conjugate vaccine. Nanomedicine (Lond) 2012; 7(5): 651-62. [http://dx.doi.org/10.2217/nnm.11.151] [PMID: 22630149]

[62] Yu M, Jambhrunkar S, Thorn P, Chen J, Gu W, Yu C. Hyaluronic acid modified mesoporous silica nanoparticles for targeted drug delivery to CD44-overexpressing cancer cells. Nanoscale 2013; 5(1): 178-83. [http://dx.doi.org/10.1039/C2NR32145A] [PMID: 23076766]

[63] Xia T, Kovochich M, Liong M, Meng H, Kabehie S, George S, *et al.* Polyethyleneimine coating enhances the cellular uptake of mesoporous silica nanoparticles and allows safe delivery of siRNA and DNA Constructs. ACS Nano 2009; 3(10): 3273-86. [http://dx.doi.org/10.1021/nn900918w]

[64] He X-x, Wang K, Tan W, Liu B, Lin X, He C, *et al.* Bioconjugated nanoparticles for dna protection from cleavage. J American Chem Soc 2003; 125(24): 7168-9. [http://dx.doi.org/10.1021/ja034450d]

[65] Mody KT, Popat A, Mahony D, Cavallaro AS, Yu C, Mitter N. Mesoporous silica nanoparticles as antigen carriers and adjuvants for vaccine delivery. Nanoscale 2013; 5(12): 5167-79. [http://dx.doi.org/10.1039/c3nr00357d] [PMID: 23657437]

[66] Al-Deen FN, Selomulya C, Ma C, Coppel RL. Superparamagnetic nanoparticle delivery of DNA vaccine. Methods Mol Biol 2014; 1143: 181-94. [http://dx.doi.org/10.1007/978-1-4939-0410-5_12] [PMID: 24715289]

[67] Al-Deen FN, Ho J, Selomulya C, Ma C, Coppel R. Superparamagnetic nanoparticles for effective delivery of malaria DNA vaccine. Langmuir 2011; 27(7): 3703-12. [http://dx.doi.org/10.1021/la104479c] [PMID: 21361304]

[68] Li Z, Liu Z, Yin M, Yang X, Ren J, Qu X. Combination delivery of antigens and CpG by lanthanides-based core-shell nanoparticles for enhanced immune response and dual-mode imaging. Adv Healthc Mater 2013; 2(10): 1309-13. [http://dx.doi.org/10.1002/adhm.201200364] [PMID: 23526798]

[69] Ribeiro AM, Souza AC, Amaral AC, *et al.* Nanobiotechnological approaches to delivery of DNA vaccine against fungal infection. J Biomed Nanotechnol 2013; 9(2): 221-30. [http://dx.doi.org/10.1166/jbn.2013.1491] [PMID: 23627048]

[70] Vyas SP, Kannan ME, Jain S, Mishra V, Singh P. Design of liposomal aerosols for improved delivery of rifampicin to alveolar macrophages. Int J Pharm 2004; 269(1): 37-49. [http://dx.doi.org/10.1016/j.ijpharm.2003.08.017] [PMID: 14698575]

[71] Vyas SP, Quraishi S, Gupta S, Jaganathan KS. Aerosolized liposome-based delivery of amphotericin B to alveolar macrophages. Int J Pharm 2005; 296(1-2): 12-25. [http://dx.doi.org/10.1016/j.ijpharm.2005.02.003] [PMID: 15885451]

[72] Joseph A, Itskovitz-Cooper N, Samira S, *et al.* A new intranasal influenza vaccine based on a novel

polycationic lipid--ceramide carbamoyl-spermine (CCS) I. Immunogenicity and efficacy studies in mice. Vaccine 2006; 24(18): 3990-4006.
[http://dx.doi.org/10.1016/j.vaccine.2005.12.017] [PMID: 16516356]

[73] Postma NS, Hermsen CC, Zuidema J, Eling WMC. Plasmodium vinckei: optimization of desferrioxamine B delivery in the treatment of murine malaria. Experimental Parasitology 1998; 89(3): 323-30.

[74] Christensen D, Korsholm KS, Rosenkrands I, Lindenstrøm T, Andersen P, Agger EM. Cationic liposomes as vaccine adjuvants. Expert Rev Vaccines 2007; 6(5): 785-96.
[http://dx.doi.org/10.1586/14760584.6.5.785] [PMID: 17931158]

[75] McNeil SE, Perrie Y. Gene delivery using cationic liposomes. Expert Opinion on Therapeutic Patents 2006; 16(10): 1371-82.
[http://dx.doi.org/10.1517/13543776.16.10.1371]

[76] Alving CR, Beck Z, Matyas GR, Rao M. Liposomal adjuvants for human vaccines. Expert Opin Drug Deliv 2016; 13(6): 807-16.
[http://dx.doi.org/10.1517/17425247.2016.1151871] [PMID: 26866300]

[77] Tyagi RK, Garg NK, Sahu T. Vaccination strategies against malaria: novel carrier(s) more than a tour de force. J Control Release Soc 2012; 162(1): 242-54.
[PMID: 22564369]

[78] Thomas C, Rawat A, Hope-Weeks L, Ahsan F. Aerosolized PLA and PLGA nanoparticles enhance humoral, mucosal and cytokine responses to hepatitis B vaccine. Mol Pharm 2011; 8(2): 405-15.
[http://dx.doi.org/10.1021/mp100255c] [PMID: 21189035]

[79] Diwan M, Tafaghodi M, Samuel J. Enhancement of immune responses by co-delivery of a CpG oligodeoxynucleotide and tetanus toxoid in biodegradable nanospheres. J Control Release Soc 2002; 85(1-3): 247-62.
[http://dx.doi.org/10.1016/S0168-3659(02)00275-4] [PMID: 12480329]

[80] Manish M, Rahi A, Kaur M, Bhatnagar R, Singh S. A single-dose PLGA encapsulated protective antigen domain 4 nanoformulation protects mice against Bacillus anthracis spore challenge. PloS One 2013; 8(4): e61885.
[http://dx.doi.org/10.1371/journal.pone.0061885] [PMID: 23637922]

[81] Demento SL, Cui W, Criscione JM, *et al.* Role of sustained antigen release from nanoparticle vaccines in shaping the T cell memory phenotype. Biomaterials 2012; 33(19): 4957-64.
[http://dx.doi.org/10.1016/j.biomaterials.2012.03.041] [PMID: 22484047]

[82] Lima VM, Bonato VL, Lima KM, Dos Santos SA, Dos Santos RR, Gonçalves ED, *et al.* Role of trehalose dimycolate in recruitment of cells and modulation of production of cytokines and NO in tuberculosis. Infect Immun 2001; 69(9): 5305-12.
[http://dx.doi.org/10.1128/IAI.69.9.5305-5312.2001] [PMID: 11500399]

[83] Hasegawa K, Noguchi Y, Koizumi F, Uenaka A, Tanaka M, Shimono M, *et al. In vitro* stimulation of CD8 and CD4 T cells by dendritic cells loaded with a complex of cholesterol-bearing hydrophobized pullulan and NY-ESO-1 protein: Identification of a new HLA-DR15-binding CD4 T-cell epitope. Clinical Cancer Res: An Official J American Association for Cancer Res 2006; 12(6): 1921-7.
[PMID: 16551878]

[84] Li P, Luo Z, Liu P, Gao N, Zhang Y, Pan H, *et al.* Bioreducible alginate-poly(ethylenimine) nanogels as an antigen-delivery system robustly enhance vaccine-elicited humoral and cellular immune responses. Journal of Controlled Release: Official J Controlled Release Society 2013; 168(3): 271-9.
[PMID: 23562637]

[85] Honda-Okubo Y, Saade F, Petrovsky N. Advax™, a polysaccharide adjuvant derived from delta inulin, provides improved influenza vaccine protection through broad-based enhancement of adaptive immune responses. Vaccine 2012; 30(36): 5373-81.
[http://dx.doi.org/10.1016/j.vaccine.2012.06.021] [PMID: 22728225]

[86] Saade F, Honda-Okubo Y, Trec S, Petrovsky N. A novel hepatitis B vaccine containing Advax™, a polysaccharide adjuvant derived from delta inulin, induces robust humoral and cellular immunity with minimal reactogenicity in preclinical testing. Vaccine 2013; 31(15): 1999-2007. [PMID: 23306367]

[87] Götze O, Müller-Eberhard HJ. The c3-activator system: an alternate pathway of complement activation. J Exp Med 1971; 134(3): 90-108. [http://dx.doi.org/10.1084/jem.134.3.90] [PMID: 19867385]

[88] Zhao K, Chen G, Shi XM, *et al.* Preparation and efficacy of a live newcastle disease virus vaccine encapsulated in chitosan nanoparticles. PLoS One 2012; 7(12): e53314. [http://dx.doi.org/10.1371/journal.pone.0053314] [PMID: 23285276]

[89] Borges O, Cordeiro-da-Silva A, Tavares J, Santarém N, de Sousa A, Borchard G, *et al.* Immune response by nasal delivery of hepatitis B surface antigen and codelivery of a CpG ODN in alginate coated chitosan nanoparticles. Euro J Pharma Biopharma 2008; 69(2): 405-16. [http://dx.doi.org/10.1016/j.ejpb.2008.01.019] [PMID: 18364251]

[90] Feng G, Jiang Q, Xia M, *et al.* Enhanced immune response and protective effects of nano-chitosa--based DNA vaccine encoding T cell epitopes of Esat-6 and FL against *Mycobacterium tuberculosis* infection. PLoS One 2013; 8(4): e61135. [http://dx.doi.org/10.1371/journal.pone.0061135] [PMID: 23637790]

[91] Pawar D, Mangal S, Goswami R, Jaganathan KS. Development and characterization of surface modified PLGA nanoparticles for nasal vaccine delivery: effect of mucoadhesive coating on antigen uptake and immune adjuvant activity. Eur J Pharm Biopharm 2013; 85(3 Pt A): 550-9. [http://dx.doi.org/10.1016/j.ejpb.2013.06.017] [PMID: 23831265]

[92] Sonaje K, Chuang EY, Lin KJ, *et al.* Opening of epithelial tight junctions and enhancement of paracellular permeation by chitosan: microscopic, ultrastructural, and computed-tomographic observations. Mol Pharm 2012; 9(5): 1271-9. [http://dx.doi.org/10.1021/mp200572t] [PMID: 22462641]

[93] de Titta A, Ballester M, Julier Z, Nembrini C, Jeanbart L, van der Vlies AJ, *et al.* Nanoparticle conjugation of CpG enhances adjuvancy for cellular immunity and memory recall at low dose. Proc Natl Acad Sci USA. 19902-7. [http://dx.doi.org/10.1073/pnas.1313152110]

[94] Mohammed MA, Syeda JTM, Wasan KM, Wasan EK. An Overview of chitosan nanoparticles and its application in non-parenteral drug delivery. Pharmaceutics 2017; 9(4): E53. [http://dx.doi.org/10.3390/pharmaceutics9040053] [PMID: 29156634]

[95] Hora MS, Rana RK, Nunberg JH, Tice TR, Gilley RM, Hudson ME. Controlled release of interleukin-2 from biodegradable microspheres. Bio/technology (Nature Publishing Company). 1990; 8(8): 755-8. [PMID: 1366902] [http://dx.doi.org/10.1038/nbt0890-755]

[96] Melissen PM, van Vianen W, Bidjai O, van Marion M, Bakker-Woudenberg IA. Free *versus* liposome-encapsulated muramyl tripeptide phosphatidylethanolamide (MTPPE) and interferon-y (IFN-y) in experimental infection with Listeria monocytogenes. Biotherapy 1993; 6(2): 113-24. [http://dx.doi.org/10.1007/BF01877424] [PMID: 8398570]

[97] Killion JJ, Fishbeck R, Bar-Eli M, Chernajovsky Y. Delivery of interferon to intracellular pathways by encapsulation of interferon into multilamellar liposomes is independent of the status of interferon receptors. Cytokine 1994; 6(4): 443-9. [http://dx.doi.org/10.1016/1043-4666(94)90069-8] [PMID: 7948753]

[98] Ha S-J, Park S-H, Kim H-J, *et al.* Enhanced immunogenicity and protective efficacy with the use of interleukin-12-encapsulated microspheres plus AS01B in tuberculosis subunit vaccination. Infect Immun 2006; 74(8): 4954-9.

[http://dx.doi.org/10.1128/IAI.01781-05] [PMID: 16861689]

[99] Dowling DJ, Scott EA, Scheid A, *et al.* Toll-like receptor 8 agonist nanoparticles mimic immunomodulating effects of the live BCG vaccine and enhance neonatal innate and adaptive immune responses. J Allergy Clin Immunol 2017; 140(5): 1339-50. [http://dx.doi.org/10.1016/j.jaci.2016.12.985] [PMID: 28343701]

[100] Moradi B, Sankian M, Amini Y, Meshkat Z. Construction of a novel DNA vaccine candidate encoding an hspx-ppe44-esxv fusion antigen of mycobacterium tuberculosis. Rep Biochem Mol Biol 2016; 4(2): 89-97. [PMID: 27536702]

[101] Xue T, Stavropoulos E, Yang M, *et al.* RNA encoding the MPT83 antigen induces protective immune responses against *Mycobacterium tuberculosis* infection. Infect Immun 2004; 72(11): 6324-9. [http://dx.doi.org/10.1128/IAI.72.11.6324-6329.2004] [PMID: 15501761]

[102] Romalde JL, Luzardo-Alvárez A, Ravelo C, Toranzo AE, Blanco-Méndez J. Oral immunization using alginate microparticles as a useful strategy for booster vaccination against fish lactoccocosis. Aquaculture 2004; 236(1): 119-29. [http://dx.doi.org/10.1016/j.aquaculture.2004.02.028]

[103] Vetro M, Safari D, Fallarini S, *et al.* Preparation and immunogenicity of gold glyco-nanoparticles as antipneumococcal vaccine model. Nanomedicine (Lond) 2017; 12(1): 13-23. [http://dx.doi.org/10.2217/nnm-2016-0306] [PMID: 27879152]

[104] Qi M, Zhang XE, Sun X, Zhang X, Yao Y, Liu S, *et al.* Intranasal nanovaccine confers homo- and hetero-subtypic influenza protection. Small (Weinheim an der Bergstrasse, Germany) 2018; 14(13): e1703207. [PMID: 29430819]

[105] Sawaengsak C, Mori Y, Yamanishi K, Mitrevej A, Sinchaipanid N. Chitosan nanoparticle encapsulated hemagglutinin-split influenza virus mucosal vaccine. AAPS PharmSciTech 2014; 15(2): 317-25. [http://dx.doi.org/10.1208/s12249-013-0058-7] [PMID: 24343789]

[106] Figueiredo L, Cadete A, Gonçalves LM, Corvo ML, Almeida AJ. Intranasal immunisation of mice against Streptococcus equi using positively charged nanoparticulate carrier systems. Vaccine 2012; 30(46): 6551-8. [http://dx.doi.org/10.1016/j.vaccine.2012.08.050] [PMID: 22947139]

[107] Khatri K, Goyal AK, Gupta PN, Mishra N, Vyas SP. Plasmid DNA loaded chitosan nanoparticles for nasal mucosal immunization against hepatitis B. Int J Pharm 2008; 354(1-2): 235-41. [http://dx.doi.org/10.1016/j.ijpharm.2007.11.027] [PMID: 18182259]

[108] Ai W, Yue Y, Xiong S, Xu W. Enhanced protection against pulmonary mycobacterial challenge by chitosan-formulated polyepitope gene vaccine is associated with increased pulmonary secretory IgA and gamma-interferon(+) T cell responses. Microbiol Immunol 2013; 57(3): 224-35. [http://dx.doi.org/10.1111/1348-0421.12027] [PMID: 23489083]

[109] Meerak J, Wanichwecharungruang SP, Palaga T. Enhancement of immune response to a DNA vaccine against *Mycobacterium tuberculosis* Ag85B by incorporation of an autophagy inducing system. Vaccine 2013; 31(5): 784-90. [http://dx.doi.org/10.1016/j.vaccine.2012.11.075] [PMID: 23228812]

CHAPTER 11

Conclusion

Abstract: From the last half of the century, scientists are developing nanoparticles for a wide variety of applications. Novel synthesis methods are explored to make them ideal for medical applications. They may be used for the detection of biological or chemical substances for the diagnosis of many disease conditions. Moreover, drugs are also delivered through nanoparticles to the target organ. Further, RNAi therapy is also supported by nanoparticles that help in the delivery of siRNA/shRNA/miRNA to the target site. DNA molecules are also conjugated with nanoparticles for gene therapy. Other than drug or gene therapy, antigens and other immunomodulators are also delivered through nanoparticles to enhance the immune response. Different vaccination strategies are also followed through nanoparticles for increased immunostimulation.

Keywords: Bioavailability, Biotechnology, Biosensing, Carbon nanoparticle, Drug delivery, Electrospraying, Gold nanoparticle, Inorganic nanoparticle, miRNA, Nanoparticle, Nanomedicine, Nanotechnology, Nanodiagnostic, Nanocarriers, Organic nanoparticle, Polymeric nanoparticle, Silver nanoparticle, siRNA, shRNA, Theranostic.

From last half of the century, researchers are developing nanoparticles in different formulations. Since the inception, scientists continuously exploring novel synthesis methods that may be fabricated depending upon the desired applications. Nanoparticles with ideal size and physiochemical properties depending upon their uses may be synthesized with already available methods such as, physical, chemical and biological synthesis methods. Nano technology is now in forefront as they have enormous potential in drug delivery and nanomedicines. Precise size and surface chemistry are the key characteristics that should be kept in mind during the synthesis. Selection of appropriate synthesis method is the key concern for optimization of size, toxicity, drug release profile, potential target, cost-effectiveness, *etc.* Electrospraying is a growing dry technology for designing polymeric nanoparticles without using toxic chemicals. The nanoformations synthesized using electrospraying may incorporate drugs/ biomolecules /growth factors that are useful in drug delivery, biosensors, tissue engineering, *etc.* moreover, electrospraying may be explored more for the

Rituparna Acharya

production of ceramic and metallic nanoparticles. Bimetallic nanoparticles have antibacterial property in contrast with the monometallic nanoparticles.

Nanoparticles may also be used for the detection system for biological and chemical targets. They provide a platform for encapsulation or incorporation of a wide variety of molecules that help in the diagnosis of disease conditions. In many sensor development applications, nanoparticles improve the selectivity and sensitivity of the assay in comparison with the conventional diagnostic methods. This nanodiagnostic technique is a low cost, rapid, easy and multiplexed identification method for biomarkers such as genes and proteins. Continuous optimization of the parameters of the nanoparticles is necessary to make them suitable for clinical use. Special effort is necessary for the development of efficient sensor that may detect target molecules from body fluid such as blood, serum urine samples. Surface of the nanoparticle may be engineered to utilize for recognition by double-stranded DNA, antibody–antigen, and aptamer–analyte interactions.

Further, nanoparticles are novel transporters that have undergone recent advancement in the delivery of drug molecules in controlled release method. Drug delivery using nanoparticles help in reducing the side effects and dosage in comparison with bare drug used in disease conditions. Three main categories of nanoparticles like inorganic, organic and polymeric are employed as drug delivery vehicle. The physiochemical properties of these nanoparticles may be tailor-made to make them biocompatible and bioavailable to the tissue structure. Synergistic action of diagnosis and therapy of these nanoparticles are known as theranostic application. The optimum size, surface structure, physical and chemical characteristics of the nanoparticles help in the targeted delivery of the drugs to the target organ. Although, a wide variety of nanoparticles are invented but the microenvironment of the biological system often influences the effective delivery of the drug molecules. The drawbacks of the use of nanocarriers are still there that limit the absorption and frequent injection to the patient. Therefore, detailed inspection of the microenvironment of the diseased tissue is of utmost importance before using these delivery vehicles. The new therapeutic regime will develop fully only when the tissue microenvironment will be studied in its fullest potential.

In this book, we have discussed the molecular mechanism of the conjugation of DNA with nanoparticles. DNA bound with gold, silver, carbon, *etc.* nanoparticles have a wide variety of applications in biological science and nanobiotechnology. Clear understanding of the mechanism of binding DNA with nanoparticles is necessary for their application in clinical diagnosis and therapy. However, the use of these nanoconjugates has raised concern of nanotoxicity and off-target side effects. DNA-nanoparticle conjugates have long-term goal in diagnosis and therapy. The main advantage of using encapsulated nanoparticles is to overcome the toxicity and for making them biocompatible.

From their invention, siRNAs have been pursued for their easy modification, high specificity, and unlimited therapeutic applications. But these molecules are highly unstable in blood vascular system. So, there is a need for designing an administering system for the delivery of siRNAs. Development of a wide variety of nanoparticles is necessary to overcome these hurdles to deliver them in the systemic circulation. They are proved to be worthy and widely recognized delivery vehicle of siRNAs. However, much research is the need of the hour for their application in curing diseases. The dynamic property of nanoparticles is influenced by the healthy and unhealthy biofluids, although much research is needed.

Another RNAi therapy is through shRNAs. Before becoming a standard procedure, shRNAs have to face number of challenges that need to be overcome. Proper targeted delivery is needed to overcome the off-target side effects that will make this approach promising in this field. Susceptibility for enzymatic degradation of these RNA molecules makes them difficult for their use as therapeutics. shRNA-nanoparticle conjugates have overcome these challenges and some of them are in clinical trial phase.

miRNAs are another type of RNAi therapeutic method. Several miRNA-nanoparticle based delivery systems have been invented for the treatment of number of diseases. Nanoparticles protect the miRNAs from degradation and inhibit the immune responses triggered by them. Recent researches have invented nanoparticles with high loading capacity that may carry the payload and deliver them on the site. New delivery vehicles must be invented to increase the half-life of the miRNA and make them bioavailable. Deeper understanding of the biological function is of utmost importance to make this therapy applicable in clinical use.

Along with the RNAi therapy, nanoparticles are used for immune modulations. Proper understanding of our immune system is important so that we can modulate it depending on our need. Manipulation of our immune system in molecular and cellular level is through nanoparticles in conjugation with immunostimulators leading to dramatic advancement in molecular medicine. In this book, we have discussed the types of immunostimulators that are conjugated with nanoparticles to enhance their efficacy.

Different types of nanoparticles have been discussed in this book that offer advantages over the traditional vaccines. The conventional vaccines use the whole microbes live or dead to elicit an immune response. However, these antigens may evoke poor immune response and thus an adjuvant is necessary to boost the immunostimulation. Nanoparticles in this respect deliver the antigens to the target site and thus evoke immunostimulation in a better way. In this book, we have discussed the variety of immunostimulators and their conjugates with nanoparticles.

This book has comprehensively covered the use of nanoparticles in medicine. We have discussed the synthesis method of nanoparticles, along with drug delivery, gene therapy, immunotherapy and vaccination strategies using nanoparticles.

Glossary

AA Anisamide

AD Adamantane

AIDS Acquired immune deficiency syndrome

ALT Serum alanine transferase

apoB Apolipoprotein B

apoE Apolipoprotein E

APP Amyloid precursor protein

AR Androgen receptor

AST Aspartate transaminase

ATTR Tranthyretin mediated amyloidosis

BMDC Bone marrow-derived dendritic cells

B-PEI Branched polyethylenimine

Ccnd1 Cyclin D1

CD Cyclodextrins

CDP Cyclodextrin-containing polycations

CH-HG Chitosan hydrogel

cLNPs Cationic LNPs

Cls Cationic liposomes

CML Chronic myeloid leukemis

CPMN Cell-penetrating magnetic nanoparticle

CPN Conjugated polymer nanoparticle

CPP Cell-penetrating peptide

CTX Chlorotoxin

DAN Copaminergic neuronal

DC Cendritic cells

DMAE N N-dimethylaminoethyl

DOPC Dioleoyl phosphatidylcholine

DOPE Dioleoylphosphatidylethanolaminev

Dox Doxorubicin

dsiRNAs Dicer substrate siRNAs

EDA Ethylene diamine

EGFP Enhanced green fluorescent protein

EHCO N-(1-aminoethyl)iminobis[N-(oleicyl-cysteinyl-histinyl- 1-aminoethyl) Propionamide]
ERK Extracellular signal-regulated kinase
FAK Focal adhesion kinase
f-MWNT Aminofunctionalized multiwalled carbon nanotubes
Gal-LipoNP Galactose-conjugated liposome nanoparticle
GAPDH Glyceraldehyde 3-phosphate dehydrogenase
GBMs Glioblastomas
GFP Green fluorescent protein
HA Hyaluronic acid
HbsAg Hepatitis B virus surface antigen
HDL High density lipoproteins
HIV Human immune deficiency virus
HMDA Hexamethylenediamine
HSP47 Heat shock protein 47
HTFs Human Tenon's fibroblasts
ICV Intracerebroventricular
iLNPs Ionizable LNPs
IV Intravenous
LCP Lipid/calcium/ phosphate
LDLc LDL cholesterol
LesiRNA Liposome-entrapped siRNA
LFA-1 Lymphocyte function Associated antigen-1
LNP Lipid nanoparticles
LODER Local drug elute R
LPD-I Cataionic liposome-polycation-DNA
LPD-II Anionic liposome- polycation-DNA
L-PEI Linear PEI
LPH Liposome-polycation-hyaluronic acid
L-PLA Poly (L-lactic acid)
MCD Mono-cationic detergent
MDR Multiple drug resistance
MEND Multifunctional envelope-type nano device
MFC Multifunctional carrier
MnMEIO Manganese-doped magnetism-engineered iron oxide
mRNA Messenger ribonucleic acid

MRTF	Myocardin-related transcription factor
MSC	Mesenchymal stem cell
MSN	Mesoporous silica nanoparticles
NB	Neuroblastoma
NgR	Nogo receptor
NP	Nanoparticle
NS	Nanoshell
ODN	Oligodeoxynucleotides
PAMAMPEG PLL	Poly(amido amine)-poly(ethylene glycol)-poly-L-lysine
PAMAM	Poly (amidoamine)
pArg	Poly-arginine
PBAE	Poly (β-amino ester)
PCL	Poly(epsilon-caprolactone)
PCSK9	Proprotein convertase subtilisin/kexin type 9
PDDA	Poly(diallyldimethylammonium) chloride
PDEAEMA	Poly (2-(diethylamino)ethylmethacrylate)
PDMAEMA	Poly (N, N-dimethylaminoethyl methacrylate)
PEC	Polyelectrolyte complex
PEG	Polyethylene glycol
PEI-	Polyethylenimine
PEO-PbAE	Poly (ethylene oxide)-modi Wed poly(beta-amino ester)
P-gp	P-glycoprotein
PIC	Polyion complex
PKN3	Protein kinase N3
PLGA	Poly (lactic-co-glycolic acid)
Plk1	Polo-like kinase 1
PLL	Poly (L) lysine peptide
pLys	Polylysine
PPD	PEG-peptide-DOPE
PPI	Propyleneimine
PRX	Polyrotaxanes
pSi	Nanoporous silicon particle
PTGS	Posttranscriptional gene silencing
PTX	Paclitaxel

QR Quantum rod
RA Rheumatoid arthritis
RFP Red fluorescent protein
RGD-CH-NP Arg-Gly-Asp-chitosan nanoparticle
rHDL Reconstituted HDL
RISC RNA-induced silencing complex
RNAi RNA interference
RRM2 Ribonucleotide reductase subunit M2
scFv Single-chain antibody fragment
siRNA Small interference ribonucleic acid
SLN Solid lipid nanoparticle
SNALP Stable nucliec acid-lipid particle
SR-B1 Scavenger receptor type B1
STAT3 Signal transducer and activator of transcription 3
STR-H8 Stearylated-octahistidine
STR-R8 Stearylated octaarginine
SWNT Single walled carbon nanotube
TDFs Tumor-derived factors
TGS Transcriptional gene silencing
THCO 1 4,7-triazanonylimino-bis[N-(oleicyl-cysteinyl-histinyl)-1aminoethyl) propionamide]
TNF-R Tumour necrosis factor-receptor
TNFα Tumor necrosis factor-α
TTR Transthyretin
UCN Upconversion nanoparticles
VEGF R2 vascular endothelial growth factor receptor-2
VEGF Vascular endothelial growth factor
WT1 Wilms' tumor gene 1

SUBJECT INDEX

A

Absorption 44, 86, 155, 168
  intestinal 86
Acid(s) 23, 24, 43, 46, 45, 57, 70, 71, 119, 123, 125, 136, 139, 141, 142, 143, 152, 158
  deoxyribonucleic 70
  folic 139
  lactic 57
  lactic-co-glycolic 136, 141, 143
  nucleic 23, 24, 43, 45, 71, 76, 125, 136, 152, 158
  polyacrylic 123
  single stranded ribonucleic 119
  uric 46
Acquired immune deficiency syndrome (AIDS) 60, 152, 153
Actinomycetes 23
Adipogenesis 106
Advantages and disadvantages 10, 11, 12, 13, 14, 15, 16, 17, 18, 19, 20, 21, 22, 23, 24, 25
  of biogenic synthesis 24, 25
  of co-precipitation method 10
  of CVD and CVS method 16
  of electrospraying method 22
  of flame spray pyrolysis method 21
  of high energy ball milling 18
  of hydrothermal technique 13
  of inert gas condensation 19
  of laser pyrolysis method 20
  of melt blending 23
  of microemulsion method 12
  of microwave 15
  of PECVD method 17
  of Physical vapor deposition method 19
  of polyol synthesis method 14
  of sol-gel method 11
Agents 12, 45, 73, 93, 123, 142, 155
  antitumor 73
  chelating 45
  immune modulatory 155
  photothermal 142
  potent anticancer 123
  theranostic 93
  triggering 12
Androgen receptor (AR) 105, 107
Angiogenesis 104, 124
Antibodies 41, 51, 62, 64, 71, 135, 138, 139, 140, 158, 168
  anti-HER2 140
Antigen(s) 4, 41, 135, 136, 137, 140, 152, 153, 154, 155, 156, 157, 158, 167, 168, 170
  bacterial 156
  delivery 4, 136
  expressing tumors 140
  immunogenic 158
  immunogenic melanoma 137
  peptide 156
  protein 156
  release 154
  transcribe fusion 158
  virus 157
Antiretroviral therapy 60
Antisense oligonucleotide technology 119
Anti-thymidylate synthase 106
Antitumor 138, 139, 140
  activity 139
  effect 138
  memory, produced 139
Apoptosis 91, 103, 104, 105, 125
  induced cellular 105
  neural 104
  tumor cell 103
Autophagosomes 137

B

Bacterial 23, 24, 25, 62, 102
  cellulose (BC) 62
  magnetosomes 102
Biogenic synthesis 23, 24, 25

Biosensing 75
application 75
assays 75
Blood 58, 60, 73, 83, 85, 121
brain barrier (BBB) 58, 60, 83, 85
coagulation 73
vascular system 121
Brain glioma cells 125
Brownian motion 12

C

Cancer 26, 27, 28, 57, 59, 63, 64, 102, 103, 104, 105, 106, 107, 123, 124, 135, 138, 139, 140, 141, 143
cell proliferation 123
colon 105
colorectal 123
gastric 102, 103
growth 102, 104
immunotherapy 139, 140, 143
macular degenerationand 104
metastatic 138
neck 141
ovarian 103, 104, 105, 107, 124, 141
pancreatic 124
silica nanoparticle 107
therapeutics 26
thymic 141
treatment of 59, 64, 123
Cancer therapy 59, 62, 105, 127, 157
ovarian 105
Cellulose 57, 62
acetate 62
nanofibrills 62
Cerebral ischemia 104
Chemical vapor 7, 15, 16
synthesis (CVS) 15, 16
deposition 7
Chemical vapor deposition 8, 16
plasma-enhanced 8
method 16
Chitosan 57, 61, 77, 100, 103, 104, 106, 117, 123, 142, 152, 157
based nanoconjugate 123
coated hollow copper sulfide 142
DNA nanoconjugate 77
nanoparticles 61, 77, 100, 103, 104, 117, 152, 157
Collision 19, 18
cluster 19
Colloidal system 13
Colorimetric 39, 45, 46, 73
analysis technique 45
detection 39, 45, 46, 73
detection of miscellaneous analytes 73
Combination therapy 105, 138
Conjugate 83, 84, 86, 93, 102, 106, 118
miRNA plasmid-nanoparticle 118
shRNA nanoparticles 106
shRNA plasmid-nanoparticle 102
siRNA-nanoparticle 83, 84, 86, 93
Connective tissue growth factor (CTGF) 106, 107
Copper-based nanoparticles (CuNPs) 50
Co-precipitation 8, 10
method 8, 10
reaction 8
Cross-linked iron oxide nanoparticles 48
Cytotoxicity 57, 64, 65, 90, 104, 138

D

Damage-associated molecular patterns (DAMPs) 141
Degradation 1, 23, 100, 108, 117, 119, 125, 136, 139, 152, 153, 169
proteolysis 136
rapid 121, 139
Delayed lung metastasis 124
Delivery 60, 86, 93, 101, 102, 104, 105, 122, 123, 124, 125, 127, 128, 135, 137, 138, 153, 156
endosomal 86
of antibodies by nanoparticles 138
nanoparticle-mediated 93
Delivery vehicle 3, 57, 58, 62, 64, 83, 122, 123, 126, 127, 128, 142

advanced 83
effective 64
novel 126
Dendritic cell(s) 135, 136, 137, 139, 141, 153, 154, 155, 158
manipulation 137
surface molecule 137
targeting 137
viability 139
Density 22, 45, 49, 74
high DNA surface 74
Detection methods 2, 73
colorimetric 45
electrochemical 49
electrochemical based 49
Detection of DNA 46, 74, 75
Dextran nanoparticle 135
Diagnostic 2, 42, 48
magnetic resonance (DMR) 48
medicine 42
technique 2
Dimethyl dioctadecyl ammonium (DDA) 157
Diseases 3, 62, 126, 152, 158
autoimmune 3
chronic skin 62
genetic 3
infectious 152, 158
neurodegenerative 126
DNA 3, 24, 45, 46, 48, 49, 51, 70, 71, 72, 73, 74, 75, 76, 77, 86, 100, 124, 157, 158, 168, 169
amine-modified 75
and gold nanoparticle 72
and increased cellular uptake 74
and rna molecules 100, 158
carbon nanotube 76
chitosan nanoparticle 77
detection in chip based microarrays 75
double stranded 72, 73
gold nanoparticle conjugate 72
nanoparticle conjugates 3, 71, 169
plasmid 3, 86
probes and gold nanoparticles 46
protein complexes 24
target 74, 75
thiolated 72
vaccine 157
DNA-quantum dot(s) 75
conjugate 75
fluorophore-FRET method 75
nanoconjugates 75
nanoconjugate 75
DNAse enzymes 76
DNA-single walled carbon nanotube 76
DNA-templated copper nanoparticle 50
DNA vaccines 153, 156, 157
gold nanoparticles 156
Downstream signaling cascades 155, 158
Drugs 2, 57, 58, 59, 60, 61, 62, 64, 65, 71, 123, 141, 167, 168
anticancer 64, 73, 141
chemotherapeutic 123
hydrophobic 64
traditional 65

E

Effects 53, 59, 64, 65, 71, 105, 141
anti-metastatic 105
anti-tumor 141
super para-magnetic 64
therapeutic 65
toxic 53, 59, 71
Efficiency 44, 57, 58, 74, 105, 127, 136, 143
catalytic 74
drug release 58
Electrical devices 26
Electrocatalysis 26
Electrochemical 39, 40, 49
analysis 49
assays 49
based detection 39, 40, 49
Electromagnetic radiation 50
Electron beam 8, 19
evaporation 19
lithography 8
Electrospraying method 22
ELISA 39, 41, 42
Emission-based detection 39, 40, 41

Endocytosis 83, 154, 155
clathrin-mediated 154
Endocytosis of siRNA-nanoparticle conjugate 86
Endosomolysis 86
Energy 12, 26
storage application 26
triggering method 12
Enzymatic 73, 85, 87, 101, 108, 156, 169
actions 108
degradation 73, 85, 87, 101, 156, 169
Enzyme-linked Immunosorbant 39
Ewing's sarcoma 103

F

Fabrication 13, 16, 17, 58, 108
of drug delivery vehicle 58
of nanoparticles 13, 16, 17
techniques 108
Fat metabolism 117
Fluorescence 39, 41, 43, 44, 45, 46, 47, 51, 74, 75, 92
based detection method 41
Detection Method 41, 74
imaging 92
Linked Immunosorbent Assay 41
metal-enhanced 51
microscopy 47
resonance energy transfer (FRET) 39, 43, 44, 45, 51, 75
Focal adhesion kinase (FAK) 104, 107
FRET assays 44
Functionalized mesoporous silica (FMS) 138

G

Gel 8, 127
electrophoresis 127
processing 8
Gene(s) 1, 3, 7, 21, 64, 70, 71, 73, 74, 75, 77, 78, 83, 84, 100, 101, 103, 104, 106, 120, 122, 124, 155, 158, 167, 168, 170
fluorescent reporter 120
immune regulatory 155
regulation nanoparticles (GRN) 106
silencing 83, 100, 103, 106
therapy 1, 3, 7, 70, 71, 73, 74, 77, 78, 100, 167, 170
viral antigen encoding 158
Genomic sequences 71
Granulocyte macrophage colonystimulating factor 158

H

Hematopoietic processes 117
Hepatitis 103, 107, 157
Hepatocellular carcinoma 124, 125
Heterogeneous semiconductors 64
High 17, 43, 74
cellular uptake 74
dye-molecule labeling ratio 43
energy ball milling method transfers 17
High encapsulation 21, 22
capacity 21
efficiency 22
Human 57, 60, 101, 103
immunodeficiency virus (HIV) 57, 60
lungadenocarcinoma cells 103
periodontalligament stem cells 101
Hydrolysis 10, 11
Hydrothermal technique 7, 8, 13
Hyperthermia-assisted cancer phototherapy 26

I

Imaging 26, 27, 28, 47, 52, 70, 72, 74, 103
intravascular MR 47
magnetic resonance 26, 27, 47, 74
photo acoustic 28
photon luminescence 26
two-photon luminescence 28
Immune 140, 154, 155, 157, 158
cells 154, 155, 157, 158
inducedcytotoxic killing 140
Immune modulating 141
compounds 141

strategy 141
Immune therapy 143
Immunity 157, 158
protective 158
Immunoassays 27, 50, 74
electrochemical 50
Immunodeficiency virus 156
Immunogenic cell death (ICD) 141, 142
Immunosensors 49
Immunostimulation 139, 143, 144, 157, 170
effective 143
elucidate 144
Immunostimulatory agents 135
Infections 60, 154, 156, 157
erythrocytic-stage malaria 157
fungal 156
mycobacteria 157
Influenza virus 157
Inhibition of tumor cell proliferation 103
Inorganic material-based delivery systems 121
Instant synthesis of metals 14
Iron 26, 64
homeostasis 64
nanoparticle biomedical applications 26

L

Lanthanides nanoparticles 27
Laser pyrolysis method 20
Ligands, dendritic cell surface 137
Light microscope 52
Lipid 57, 62, 107, 123, 124, 137, 157
adjuvant monophosphoryl 137
based nanoconjugate 83
Lipid nanoparticle 47, 100, 102, 117, 124, 135, 140
cationic 124
multilamellar 140
solid 102
synthetic 47
Lipofectamines 119
Liposomes 47, 57, 59, 62, 93, 136, 139, 140, 156, 157
cationic 136
study stealth 139
Liquid chromatography 127
Low molecular weight chitosan (LMWC) 104
Lung cancer 102, 106, 124, 139
advanced metastatic 139
Lung tumorigenesis 103
Lymphocytes 136, 138, 139, 141, 143
tumor infiltrating 139

M

Macrophages 47, 58, 85, 136, 138, 140, 155, 158
tumor-associated 138
Macropinocytosis 155
Magnetic 26, 27, 39, 40, 46, 47, 48, 52, 74, 83, 88, 93, 100, 101, 102, 107
and electrical applications 26
based detection 39, 40, 47
nanoparticles 46, 47, 48, 74, 83, 88, 93, 100, 101, 102, 107
resonance imaging (MRI) 26, 27, 39, 47, 52, 74
Magnetic fields 15, 64, 65, 88
oscillating 15
transfection 88
Melanoma-associated epitope 137
Metal enhanced fluorescence (MEF) 39, 50, 51
Microbes 4, 170
killed 4
live attenuated 4
Microcrystalline cellulose 62
Microemulsion method 11, 12
MiRNAs 119, 120
endogenous 119
upregulating 120
Multidrug resistance cells 103
Multi drug resistance protein 106
Multiplexed identification method 168
Myeloid-derived suppressive cells (MDSCs) 138
Myocardial fibrosis treatment 106

N

Nanocrystals 62, 70, 123
  cellulose 62
Nanodiagnostic technique 168
Nanomaterials 1, 7, 11, 70, 71, 78, 108, 122, 155
  hybrid 108
  inorganic 11
  polymeric 122
Nanoparticle 21, 106, 107
  disease 106, 107
  fabrication method 21
Nanoparticles 14, 19, 25, 46, 50, 51, 64, 83, 87, 91, 105, 117, 138, 139, 140, 154, 167, 168
  copper 50
  cyclodcxtrin 91, 117
  designing polymeric 167
  fluorescent 64
  gold and silver 25, 46, 51
  hybrid 14, 19
  hydrophilic 154
  hydrophobic 154
  liposome-protamine-hyaluronic acid 139
  mannose-modified 138
  mercury selenide 50
  metal oxide 83
  monometallic 168
  peptide-conjugated PEG 105
  polystyrene 140
  quantum dote 117
  traditional medicines 87
Nature 1, 62, 86, 93, 117, 122, 123
  anionic 86, 122
  cationic 123
  dendritic 62
  dynamic 93
  fragile 1, 117
Near-infrared photodynamic therapy 27
Negligible nuclease activity 90
Neurodegeneration 102
Nonmolecular chromophores 44
Nuclear magnetic resonance (NMR) 39, 47, 48
Nucleation 8, 9, 12
  process 12
  reaction 12
  stage 8, 9
Nucleic 72, 124
  acid delivery vehicle proteins 124
  Acid detection 72

O

Oligonucleotide(s) 46, 72, 73, 74, 127, 136
  functionalized gold nanoparticle 45
  probe 74
  detecting DNA 75
Optical imaging 52
Organic 15, 61, 102, 152, 156
  nanoconjugates 102, 152, 156
  polymer based nanocarriers 61
  synthetic method 15
Organic nanoparticle 123, 143
  based delivery of miRNA and anti-miRNA 123
  liposomal nanoparticles 143
Organogenesis 117
Osteosarcoma 102
Ostwald ripening procedure 9

P

Parkinson's disease 102, 107
Pathogen associated molecular patterns (PAMPs) 136, 158
PEG-PLA nanoparticles 140
PEGylated 77, 139
  liposome encapsulating 139
  nanoparticle 77
Penta fluorophenyl methacrylate 143
Peptide based nanoconjugate 124
Peptides 45, 71, 124, 126, 137, 142, 156
  antigenic 156
  cleavable substrate 126
  tumor antigen 137

tumor homing 142
Phagocytosis 85, 86, 140, 141
Photocatalysis 27
Photodynamic therapies 26, 141
Photolithography 8
Photoluminescence devices 27
Photothermal therapies 141
Plasma 16, 17
enhanced chemical vapor deposition (PECVD) 16
stream 17
Plasmid(s) 120, 156, 158
DNA encoding 156
expressing 120
Plasmonics-based detection 39, 40, 50
Platelet-derived growth factor (PDGF) 73, 104
Poly(b-amino ester) (PAEs) 106
Polymeric Nanoconjugates 103, 152, 157
Polymers 7, 22, 47, 58, 62, 77, 83, 86, 90, 91, 93, 123, 124, 125, 138, 139, 157
cationic 77, 86
natural 157
renewable 62
synthetic 47, 124, 125, 157
wide variety of 90, 124
Polyol synthesis method 14
Precursors 7, 8, 10, 11, 12, 14, 16, 17, 21, 120
single stranded 120
Process 88, 154
cell signaling 154
cellular transport 88
Production 10, 17, 47, 71, 91, 127, 138, 139, 142, 155, 157, 158, 168
cytokine 138, 142, 155
industrial 8
nitric oxide 157
Programmed cell death protein 140
Prokaryotic bacteria 23
Properties 7, 9, 39, 40, 48, 49, 50, 57, 58, 59, 61, 65, 71, 87, 88, 89, 90, 92, 93, 122, 123, 138, 142, 153, 159, 169
adjuvant 153, 159
antibacterial 168
biodegradable 61, 122
dynamic 93, 169
electrochemical 49
hydrophobic 59
immunogenic 159
intrinsic 65
nontoxic 122
physicochemical 58
semiconductor 123
superparamagnetic 48
theranostic 71
therapeutic 92
tunable 142
Prostate cancer 104, 105, 106, 124
cell line 104
combination therapy 105
independent 106
Protein(s) 21, 24, 43, 45, 46, 48, 51, 52, 57, 83, 103, 117, 124, 137, 156
expressions 83
synthesis 83, 103
tumor antigen 137
Pulmonary metastasis 105

Q

Quantum dot 42, 43, 44, 49, 75, 76, 83, 93, 123
fluorophores 42
nanoconjugate 123
nanoparticles 43, 44, 49, 75, 76, 83, 93

R

Radiofrequency saturation 47
Raman spectroscopy 52
Rapid analysis process 20
Reaction 8, 10, 13, 14, 15, 39, 40, 53, 58, 75, 123, 124, 154, 157
antigen-antibody 53, 58
catalytic 75
immunogenic 123, 124
immunological 154, 157
polycondensation 11
polymerase chain 39
Reactive oxygen species (ROS) 27, 142

Reduced 20, 57, 121
cytotoxicity 57
expense 20
intracellular delivery 121
Reduction 10, 14, 24, 103, 141, 156
electrochemical 10
Renal clearance 85
Repressing gene expression 121
Response 64, 85, 90, 93, 108, 136, 138, 141, 155, 157
altered cellular 64
anti-tumor immunotherapy 141
dynamic 93
elicited inflammatory 155
extended therapeutic 138
immunogenic 85
low antigenic 108
lymphocyte 136
Retinopathy 104, 107
diabetic 104, 107
RNA 100, 121, 126, 127
delivery vehicles 121
interference therapy 100
nanoparticle conjugate 126, 127
RNA-induced silencing 83, 101
complex (RISC) 83, 101
RNA molecules 1, 24, 100, 101, 117, 119, 120, 124, 126, 127, 158
large molecular weight 127
single stranded 119
RNAs 48, 57, 75, 83, 86, 100, 119, 126, 127, 152, 153
double-stranded 83
plasmid encoding 119
plasmid transcribes sponge 119
RNase enzymes 100

S

Sandwich hybridization strategy 74
Signals 2, 43, 73, 142
fluorescent 73
produced 142
Silica 45, 57, 83, 87, 122, 156
based nanoparticles 83
based biosensing method 45
mesosporous 156
Silica nanoparticles 39, 41, 43, 45, 47, 57, 64, 87, 93, 100, 102, 142, 152, 156
glutathione-depleted dendritic mesoporous 142
liposome-coated mesoporous 142
porous structure mesoporous 142
spherical mesoporous 87
Single 72, 74
DNA 72
stranded DNAs 72, 74
Sirna therapy 84, 87
SNP analysis 52
Sol-gel 7, 8, 10, 11
method 7, 8, 10, 11
procedure 11
Squamous cell carcinoma 124
Stability 21, 48, 49, 63, 64, 75, 83, 86, 87, 88, 92, 93, 117, 119, 120, 121, 126, 127
chemical 64, 92, 93
demonstrated 75
intestinal 85
intrinsic 63
low colloidal 88
mechanical 21
Substances 157, 158, 167
chemical 167
immunostimulatory 158
Suppression 104, 107, 119, 140
immune 140
Surface 1, 13, 18, 43, 48, 50, 51, 57, 59, 65, 87, 153, 167
adsorption 153
chemistry 1, 13, 43, 48, 57, 65, 87, 167
conduction electrons 50
conjugation 153
contamination 18
enhanced infrared absorption (SEIRA) 50, 51
enhanced Raman scattering (SERS) 39, 50
property of nanoparticles 59
Survivin shRNA and 104, 105
vascular endothelial growth factor 104

adamantine-paclitaxel 105
Synergistic 70, 168
action of diagnosis and therapy 168
activity 70
Synthesis 8, 15, 16, 25
bio-assisted 8
chemical vapor 15, 16
efficiency 25
Synthesis method 2, 7, 8, 11, 12, 13, 14, 15, 17, 18, 20, 21, 22, 23, 24, 89, 167
biological 167
facile 89
mediated 23
novel 167

T

Targeted 27, 158
delivery ability 158
drug delivery vehicles 27
Targeting gastric cancer cells 106
Technology 1, 7, 10, 50, 53, 119, 127
anti-miRNA oligonucleotide 119
sensing 50
Therapeutic 3, 27, 71, 84, 87, 89, 93, 102, 121, 125, 135, 137, 140
agents 125, 135
applications 3, 27, 71, 84, 87, 89, 93, 102, 121, 137
cellular engineering by nanoparticles 140
Therapy 3, 28, 88, 94, 117, 119, 135, 168, 169
cancer therapeutics Cell 28
Thrombin protein 75
Thymidylate synthase (TS) 106, 107
Thymine 72
Tissue(s) 57, 62, 65, 117, 118, 122, 124, 125, 138, 167, 168
accessibility 138
colon 125
diseased 65, 168
microenvironment 168
target disease 57
Toll-like receptor (TLR) 136, 137
Toxic 27, 167
chemicals 167
gases, removing 27
Toxicity 2, 22, 24, 50, 60, 62, 87, 88, 91, 93, 103, 107, 108, 135, 139, 140, 143, 144, 157, 167, 169
chitosan nanoparticles 103
low 50, 91, 108, 143, 144
off-target 107
reduced 22, 24, 157
systemic 143
Toxic 10, 136
liquid waste 10
shock syndrome 136
Transduction 2
methods 2
processes 2
Transfection 93, 100, 103, 119
efficient 93
Transfection efficiency 77, 125
demonstrated high 125
Transforming growth factor 103, 141
Tumor 48, 118, 137, 138, 139, 141, 142
advanced solid 139
associated macrophages (TAMs) 138
microenvironment 138
regression 137
Tumor antigen 137
peptides (TAPs) 137
Tumor cells 48, 60, 103, 137, 140, 141
apoptotic 141
proliferation 103
prostate 140
sensitizing 141
Tumor growth 102, 104, 124, 138, 139, 141, 142, 143
inhibited 139
protected 124
reduced 139
regressed 139

V

Vaccination 1, 4, 142, 152, 153, 167, 170
strategies 152, 167, 170

Vaccine 4, 152, 155, 156
delivery 4, 155, 156
development 152
Vascular 1, 83, 85, 87, 103, 104, 106, 121, 122, 126, 169
endothelial growth factor (VEGF) 103, 104, 106
endothelium 85, 87
system 1, 83, 121, 122, 126, 169

W

Waste, solid 10
Water disinfection 26

X

Xanthan gum 57, 62
Xanthomonas campestris 62

Z

Zinc oxide 27

www.ingramcontent.com/pod-product-compliance
Lightning Source LLC
LaVergne TN
LVHW070119110826
845147LV00002B/156

* 9 7 8 1 6 8 1 0 8 8 3 7 2 *